Cancer as an Initiation

C [illegible] tion

Opening to the Gifts of Cancer and Letting the the Love in

A journey of Healing, awakening to Soul Purpose and Listening to the body as a Muse

By Rachael Crow

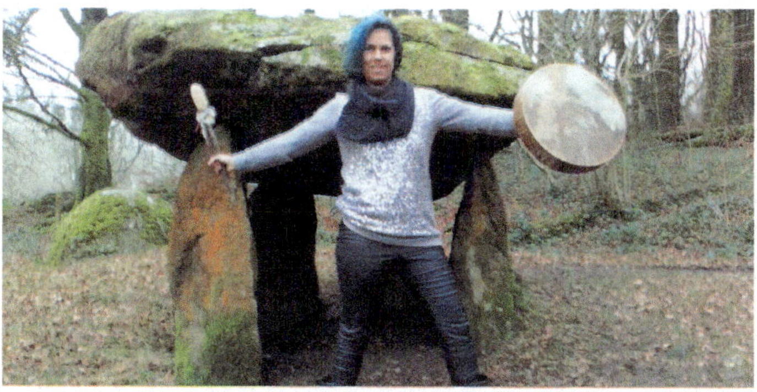

Cancer as an Initiation

First edition ISBN 978-1-3999-7257-4

Cover design by Rachael Crow and Jericho O'Neill

DISCLAIMER

This book may contain general information relating to cancer and cancer treatment. Such information is provided for informational purposes only and is not meant to be a substitute for medical advice.

You should not use the information contained herein for diagnosing a health problem or disease. You should always consult with your physician or other qualified health care professional for medical advice or information about diagnosis and treatment.

The information in this book and web resources are presented "as is, and" for educational purposes only. It is not intended as a substitute for the diagnosis, treatment, or advice of a qualified, licensed medical professional, and in no way should anyone infer that I, the author, am practicing medicine.

I recommend that you do your own independent research before using or purchasing anything.

Books by this author

Menarche: a Journey into Womanhood

Thirteen Moons: a compilation of Women's Wisdom/Women's Mysteries

Why Does Mummy Bleed?

Testimonials and praise

Rachael traverses her health recovery journey with a radical awareness that is as inspiring as it is educational.

Her story of healing has the power to shift your perspective on what's possible, and open you to a new level of appreciation for the wonder of being alive.

Lee Harris, Energy Intuitive, Musician and Channeller

Rachael's story is heroic to its core. She shows just what is possible when we look for the gifts to embrace within life's challenges, rather than the obstacles to battle against. Rachael has retained sovereignty throughout her path of healing, always choosing the medical natural protocols that felt right to her. This book is a must read for anyone with a significant health challenge looking to recover whilst remaining in control of their experience.

Andrew Kempleton, Author and Shamanic practitioner

Rachael's book is both an invitation to really step into whole bodied life, and yet also an honest powerful look into death, so taboo culturally. She is able to challenge how we receive such 'big' health information, whilst honouring every individual on their path, she shared deeply and powerfully of what is stirred in her. Her ability to live and gesture the balance of both humility and powerful decision making are an inspiration, staying true to herself and inviting us all to reflect on being here now! A book that is relevant to anyone open to initiations and healing, big and small. The healing manifesto should be put on all our walls. Gratitude and Love to Rachael, for your wisdom, courage, and commitment to truth within.

Dominique Sakoilsky, Author, Relationship therapist, Cranial sacral therapist

In her book, Rachael lays bare her own journey, embarking on a deeply personal quest to discover her true self while allowing cancer to serve as her initiator. As you immerse yourself in her words, it's as if you're right there beside her, navigating the turbulent waters of her courageous healing journey. Rachael possesses an uncanny ability to transform every obstacle into a powerful teaching moment, generously imparting these invaluable insights to her readers.

I can't help but be profoundly moved by Rachael's story, and I can confidently say that her words have ignited a profound sense of purpose within me. Her narrative invites all of us to take the reins of our health and our lives, and it's worth noting that this book should come with a warning: After reading, you will be brimming with an impassioned desire to initiate change in your life.

To Rachael, I extend my heartfelt gratitude for sharing this profoundly transformative experience with both me and the world. Your story will forever resonate within me as a beacon of strength and inspiration.

Salena Walker - Naturopath, Herbalist and Nutritionist www.salenawalker.earth

Rachael's book is must read for anyone with cancer, or with a loved one with cancer, as well as those interested in healing or a passion for initiation. This raw, honest, authentic and courageous book is testimony to the power of radical self-love and care, and a revolutionary new way of looking at cancer ~ a retelling of the story that we have all be programmed to believe.

The reader is inspired and soothed throughout by Rachael's warrior heart, and generous, supportive voice heard in every word she writes, and it feels as if she has taken us by the hand and that we can overcome any dark shadow that the world may bring to our door. Her sage advice applies to all experiences of disease and illness, and dark nights of the Soul. We can take back responsibility from the hands of others, rather than handing them over in fear, and instead connect to our intuition, the Earth (our Great Mother) and our hearts and souls for these places are the sacred spaces where true healing lives. In this, we can rewrite the stories our culture and paradigm has written in our bodies. This book is a reminder that nothing is done to us or can be done for us, rather that everything that comes into our lives is for us as a potential gift of empowerment and that we are our own saviours.

Rachael has followed a path that has taken her to the doorway of death.

Looking straight into its face and learning to be at peace with it rather than to fear it, to love it rather than fight it. She has followed in the footsteps of true initiates across time and culture.

Rachael tells us "live life as a ceremony" I suggest we all begin right away.

Penny Champ - Wild Sister Wisdom

Magic exists in those moments when we tap into our innate power….Rachael guides us into this magical realm with her writings….her musings…..her feelings….her inner knowledge of a process of initiation that unfolded to give the gift of good health…..

I left Rachael's world , those words on her pages, with a sense of power……a power of faith, a faith my own ability to health

Peta Inglesent, Innate biophile (lover of life) , Intuitive Therapist & long term Stage 4 metastatic cancer thriver.

To make choices that go against the flow of majority thought is not easy. It takes a certain self awareness to stand in the face of challenge and choose your own path. But when that path is in the collective consciousness called cancer, standing in sovereign truth is a heroic journey. Rachael is that unique soul who chose her destiny towards health in her way despite the well meaning pressures to cave into the depths of fear. She followed her inner guidance, choosing to walk both worlds, allopathic medicine and alternative. It was so refreshing to read this inspiring book that is leading the way to a new paradigm in body healing and awareness. There are those who show us how and Rachael opens her world to us in a way that is vulnerable, raw, and attainable.

As someone who has experienced stage 3 breast cancer and chose my own path to life and vitality, loving my body to wellness, I am beyond thrilled to endorse Rachel Crow's book, Cancer as an Initiation. The world needs her book but even more importantly, I needed her book. It reminded me how powerful sharing can change the world. Thank you Rachael.

Becki Koon, Best Selling Author of 20 Days Changed Everything and Breathe The Deep Waters Of Love. Energy Intuitive, Holy Fire III & Karuna Reiki Master. www.beckikoon.com

I dedicate this book to my amazing community who supported me - too many to list- this book is dedicated to ALL OF YOU!

I couldn't have done this journey without YOU ALL.

"It takes a village to heal"

Contents

Foreword by Annee Bury

Rachael is a mother of four, an accomplished spiritual and womens facilitator helping women recover from the trauma of the wounded feminine, it not surprising therefore that she was given cancer of the cervix, womb and ovaries for her own personal healing.

Diagnosed during lockdown she shares her journey through primary and secondary diagnosis, spiritual, holistic, nutritional and modern medicine and courageously making friends with death. She learns to surrender and trust her inner wisdom and steps into a life lived in trust and gifted with love.

I was one of the many women who Racheal invited to support her in her healing journey, having worked as a cancer mentor and experienced a challenging cancer diagnosis as initiation myself, we danced together with a deep soul knowing of the value and gift of this journey. She was a joy to mentor.

I feel honoured to have been asked to write the foreword for this book about her inspiring, challenging and unusual journey into healing herself.

This book is revolutionary, it turns the cancer story upside down, instead of fighting from a place of fear it is a journey into self love, self empowerment and wholeness. I have never read a cancer journey where someone dives so deeply into the unknown and reclaims her soul, her health and her life. Working and playing with the cancer journey as initiation, calling on the sacred through the power of ritual and ceremony reframes it into a journey through life, death and rebirth,

Rachaels writing style is such that she invites you to step into her life and walk alongside her and to feel and live the ups and downs of her journey whilst absorbing and learning so much along the way, this is a journey of strength and truth a journey of and for the heart. The book is riveting, inspiring, funny, painful and honest.

This book will become a life line for people diagnosed with cancer. Rachael's story is healing in itself and her generous links to resources, blogs, self healing tool box and her healing manifesto gives the reader both a menu and a recipe for their own journey through cancer and for living their future life. A must read for anyone on this healing journey.

Annee xxx

Annee Bury is someone who has extensive experience of a holistic and integrated approach to Cancer as Initiation, her expertise comes from being a nurse, a hospice and palliative care educator, a shamanic healer, a cancer mentor, a death guide and funeral celebrant as well as having had her own diagnosis of an aggressive cancer 10 years ago.

"The Body has a Super Wisdom within that is biased towards health, rather than towards disease."

The Dynamic Laws of Healing

Introduction

I recognise that my experience was different from many others, as I had already been walking the path of healing, journeying, ritual, meditation and energy work.

I wrote this book to inspire people, to help them step out of fear into love and to support them to be empowered to take their own path of healing. This isn't a book on "how to heal cancer", but how to deal with cancer. How to live authentically with cancer.

I invite you in to my life, and my journey.

Please remember that everyone has their stories about cancer, and friends who died (yep, me too- and there's a section about that- along with- how to deal with friends who find it difficult to support your choices). There are also plenty of stories of people who heal…miraculously. And I believe in miracles, because I've seen them! If you want to find out even more about healing cancer- then check out the resources page at the end of this book.

Do you have cancer? Does your friend? As you might imagine, I have a LOT of people making contact with desperate cancer stories, which is why I created this book. Ultimately, I cannot help anyone who doesn't want to help themselves, plus they also need to be FREE FROM FEAR to take the self-educated, and empowered route with cancer.

I can't help anyone apart from offer what I myself have found useful, which was a deep spiritual belief, surrender, acceptance, a wonderful support team, a deep intuition that my body would heal...and a passion that food can be our medicine.

A note on the formatting of the book; I purposely created large margins for you to make notes, (Yes, I'm encouraging you to scribble on this book) and a larger type so you can comfortably read in bed, lying on the sofa, or on the train without too much effort.

Rachael Crow 2023

Acknowledgements

To my family - especially Dorothy and Emrys who watched Mummy go from healthy warrior to poorly chemo mum. Emrys said to me recently (3 years post chemo) "Mummy, we had no idea stage 4 was the worst cancer could be, we thought it was 4/10 so we didn't think it was too bad!" I replied, "Well, it was probably best you thought that, otherwise you might have been very worried about me." Bless him.

Jericho for challenging me as only a son can do, helping me see 'outside the box'.

Tabi, I know it was hard being so far away. I'm proud of you for living your life on your terms.

Tom, who put on his stoic armour and just held me through it all- love does all it's capable of doing.

To my family and friends who were too far away (or locked down!) to help, but sent gifts, donations, and prayers- I thank you for adding to the collective field of healing.

Gratitude to C&M organics for the consistent flow of local organic food and to Team Verrico for the support towards paying.

Huge thanks to all the amazing practitioners and therapists who supported me authentically- and went beyond what they were 'allowed' to do in the scope of recommendations for cancer.

Thank you Salena, Ali and Lesley, Ed, Andy, Dominique and Louise, Lianne, Elaine, Dr Kemfen, Trevor, Eartha, Ayres, Michelle: all those whose hands were part of my healing.

Sally Light, her friendship and her own cancer journey inspired me all the way. Fly high beautiful butterfly Sally.

Lee, your meditations and music kept my vibe high even in 'scanxiety'!

David, your cancer journey and meditations gave me hope and faith.

Dr Joe and Leland- for helping me use my energy wisely and BREATHE!

Gail- your womens spiral has been a foundation- thank you for introducing me to it.

Cancerucan, THANK YOU all you guys and the weekly healing team.

Annee, my amazing 'cancer mentor'- thank you for holding me accountable and helping me through this initiation.

Jen and Ant for the hot tub party (!). Creating a community space, and being our long standing friends here in Wales.

Penny, my Red Tent/Drum sistar in Aus- thank you for your elder wisdom and friendship.

Amber, my 'cancer doula' for my early appointments- everyone needs a friend along side them.

To anyone I've forgotten, I place you in my 'community thanks'- I love you all.

Chapter 1

My hopes and intentions with this book

The biggest hope for me is that this book helps to remove fear from it's association with the word cancer. The journey I have been through with my family, (including my children seeing me and witnessing me heal from stage 4 cancer), means they have no fear of that word. As far as they are concerned, you can heal from cancer, you can heal from anything if you want to, if you are willing to surrender to the journey and give it your all.

Maybe this book will help you to develop a new story about cancer, not one that has been given to us by our society and the dominant medical paradigm; one in which we live in fear and become helpless victims and then are cured or die. So my hope is that you realise that you are a human being capable of miracles, self-knowledge and, self-love, and become empowered to listen and make your own decisions and healing choices. And most of all to learn the gift of self-love.

In our collective story of cancer = death, it's time to break that narrative. It's time to share stories of recovery, of living well with cancer, living well despite cancer! And also to understand that a major part of our healing is to make friends with death in order to heal. So perhaps this collective story can wake us up to both death and to life itself.

I want to offer you tools to guide you on your healing journey and journey of recovery. To lead you on a path less travelled.To show you how to bring joy into your life. To encourage you to listen deeply to your own wisdom, intuition, to watch for synchronicities. To allow the Divine to guide you to wellness.

There are so many protocols out there. I know how confusing and overwhelming it can be - I've been through it. What I have learned is that, ultimately, there is no single package that works. YOU have to feel in to what is right for you. You are the one that needs to make the changes. But I can energetically hold your hand. Every initiation has to be taken alone, but you can do it with support, and I can be part of your support team through this book!

I have to admit I was resistant to writing this book. I had let go of the 'cancer story' and was getting on with life. Yes, I still support people, offer a helping hand and suggestions to those who are open to change, but I wasn't seeing 'cancer support' as a new career. I was walking into my new cancer-free life. However, after doing some talks and interviews, I realised that I had walked a path less trodden, the path of seeing illness as an Initiation. So here's my story. There's so much more I could have written about, but I feel complete in this offering. You'll find plenty more on my YouTube and blog. I want to empower you, my readers, to find your path, and walk your own less trodden way. Take the s/hero's journey. You won't regret it!

Miracles and Initiation

I believe my healing came from my deep spiritual belief that I was being guided to my soul purpose, embracing surrender and acceptance. I also had a wonderful support team of therapists, along side friends and family. In Shamanic traditions, it takes a village to heal a person. I was blessed to be held by my community who encouraged me, cooked for me, took care of my children, gave me massages, reiki, foot rubs, brought me juices and smoothies, drove me to hospital appointments, sent me healing and prayed for me. I was loved well. My heart is full of gratitude for my life and my community.

Oh, and I expected a miracle- I was open to a miracle and I gave thanks every day for my miracle!

What is initiation?

From the Cambridge dictionary- https://dictionary.cambridge.org/dictionary/english/initiation

An occasion when something starts

An occasion when someone is first introduced to an activity or skill

The act of beginning something

A special ceremony or responsibility that signals the acceptance of someone into a group

https://www.merriam-webster.com/dictionary/initiation

Definition of initiation

1a : the act or an instance of initiating

b : the process of being initiated

c : the rites, ceremonies, ordeals, or instructions with which one is made a member of a sect or society or is invested with a particular function or status

2 : the condition of being initiated into some experience or sphere of activity : knowledgeableness

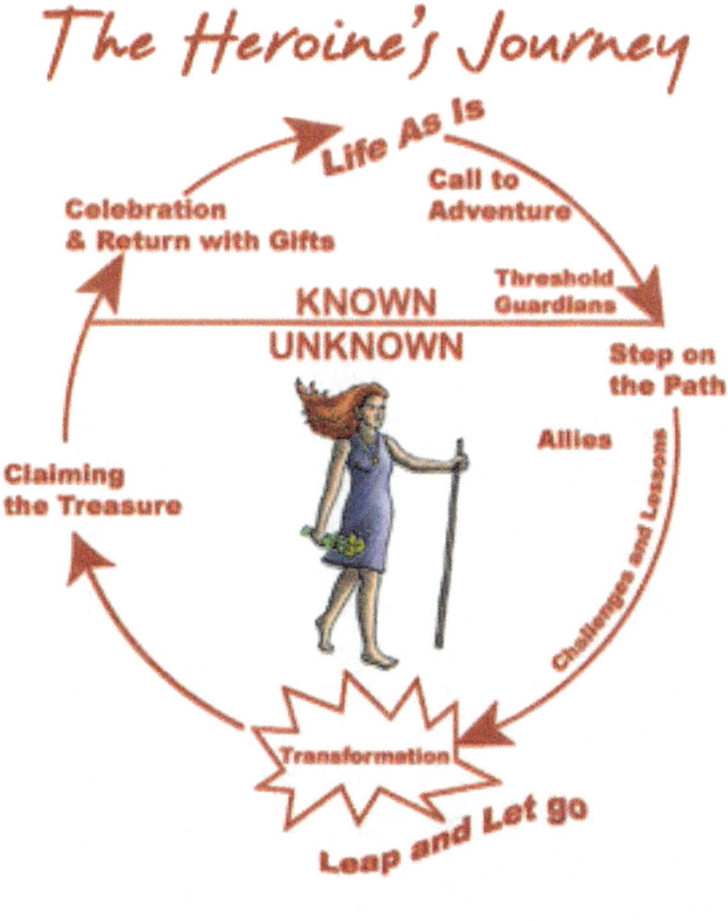

I would define initiation as a process that involves dark nights of the soul, deep questioning, challenge, rebirth- going deep into the cocoon to emerge as a butterfly! It can also be seen as the Heroines/Hero's Journey.

It's an opportunity to look into the mirror of life, and see the soul reflected back, clearly witnessing the choices we have made along our journey. A soul initiation can be our opportunity for greater awareness and clarity about life and where our path is taking us.

And when I renamed this diagnosis as an 'Initiation' I had a big sigh of relief in my body that I could do this because I know what initiation is.

I have spent most of my life working with rites of passage and initiation. This has been through ceremony, quests and challenges, in my workshops, on camps and the year- long training I have offered, including honouring a woman's life initiations (such as first blood, birth, menopause, crone/elder) and all the transitions between. So when I refer to cancer as an initiation, it was because I realised that as I had held so many girls and women on my life journey through their initiations, now it was time for me to surrender to one of the biggest initiations of all.

I believe that life gives us wake up calls, and that sometimes these are small nudges, and if we don't listen, the nudges become shoves, and the shoves become shouts and if still not heeded, shouts turn into crisis. I had quite a few things going on in my life that I knew needed changing, or totally letting go. There had been opportunities along the way for this to happen, but it was easy to stay plodding along doing the same old thing- when really my soul was nudging me for growth and adventure. I HAD to let go of the old me and allow the big changes to happen. In fact, when I stopped resisting it all became much easier than I could ever have imagined.

I also realise that whatever you put out into the world, the world will reflect back to you. So as someone holding initiations and ceremonies, it was apt in one way that life would throw me the biggest initiation of all. ***Cancer***.

For years I hadn't wanted to run my business any more. But it was something I'd built up from scratch. I'd been on the front line in my field for many years, offering menstrual work, selling cloth pads, moon sponges and cups, and writing books on rites of passages for women and girls yet my baby was almost 30 years old. The truth was, I had outgrown it, even though part of me was hanging on. When the stage 4 diagnosis came in, I knew I had to let it go. It was time to give this baby to someone else to nurture. I worked with a business coach, who helped me vision some 'new parents' for my business baby. Very soon I had an offer, and it all flowed so smoothly, I was able to let go with ease, and also trust, as I now had no idea what I would do next. What I did know was that it was time for ME to HEAL and to really allow myself to embrace this initiation fully.

Chapter 2

My Diagnosis story and awakenings around love

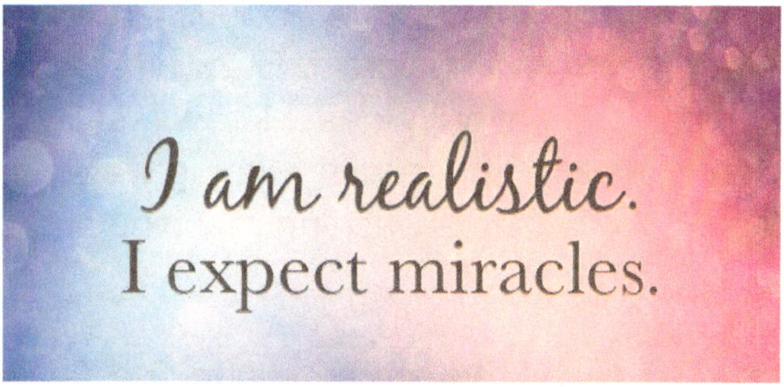

You'll find with most cancer patients they will have had some sort of stress/trauma not long before diagnosis. My story is one of those. Cutting a very long story short, I will try and condense what happened over a few years into one chapter.

My husband and I moved to west Wales in 2011 to 'live the good life'. I'd brought up my two eldest children in Bristol as a single mum, and for years had been hankering after a life in the country. When I met Tom it was one of the things we had in common. We had Dorothy in 2010, when my eldest were twenty-one and eighteen, old enough to be flying the nest, except we were the ones who flew the nest. Leaving them to rent the house we had been living in together.

When we first moved we were living in a caravan in the garden of our friends, having bought some land with Tom's parents, with a dream of living there and being self sufficient. But when I found my self pregnant at forty-one, I knew I really needed to be in a house with running water and electricity, as well as a washing machine and a bath!

Things didn't work out with the land and Toms parents, let's just say our beliefs and ways of living were too different. We rented a small cottage and I had a beautiful home birth. It wasn't long before the next idea came along, which was to buy a house and land with two other families, with the vision of attracting more families and creating an eco-community.

By this time Emrys was around two years old and Dorothy five, I was forty three and peri menopause was beginning. Migraines, insomnia and hot flushes had all kicked in, my cycle was all over the place and I was super stressed. Starting a community meant lots of meetings, a large investment of money plus trying to create business plans so we would be able to recoup some of our investment. Along side this, my husband and I were both working. I was self-employed so I was running my business, alongside juggling childcare and work. I found the added stress of the community taking its toll.

Once again we were living in a caravan (a bit bigger this time), so there was also the added pressure of all being on top of one another, this was balanced out with the beauty of the land, being able to be outside a lot helped, I had begun to have anxiety and panic attacks (which I had never experienced in my life!) so I often just lay on the earth until the anxiety passed. The balancing act continued until I got to breaking point, there were personality clashes with the other families, our marriage was under so much pressure, earning money to keep ourselves afloat while mothering, working, not sleeping, it was too much and I felt like I was going mad. I pulled back from everything and retreated into myself. I was blessed to have an amazing women's circle that I had started with Emrys was a baby and my sisters from this circle were so supportive and caring, but even with this support, I knew big changes needed to be made and I had even started saying to Tom that living in community was making me ill. Symptoms (which I thought were all perimenopause related) had begun- pain, bleeding between cycles on top of the anxiety, insomnia, migraines...

Incidentally these symptoms had nudged me to take a basic nutrition training and I felt it was important to support my body as it went though "the change" and I'm pretty sure the changes I made with my diet and lifestyle slowed down the cancer growth.

Tom was worried about the financial investment we had made and felt strongly we needed to stay and protect that, and he really wanted the children to grow up surrounded by nature. There were very few places to rent and those that were available were located in towns and not where we wanted to be. But I knew I had to leave. My intuition was screaming at me to get out, so in the end I found a place for rent through friends and left Tom and the children in the community. I was whooping with relief when I drove away with my car loaded up!

My new home was down a long track, with only a few neighbours, surrounded by trees and peace. It was a sanctuary.

Tom and I shared the parenting, taking turns having the children for a few days in the week and during weekends However while it seemed ideal, it was disrupting for the children and for the first few months I was still crying whenever they left. I missed Tom terribly. I hadn't intended our marriage to break up, I just needed my sanity back.

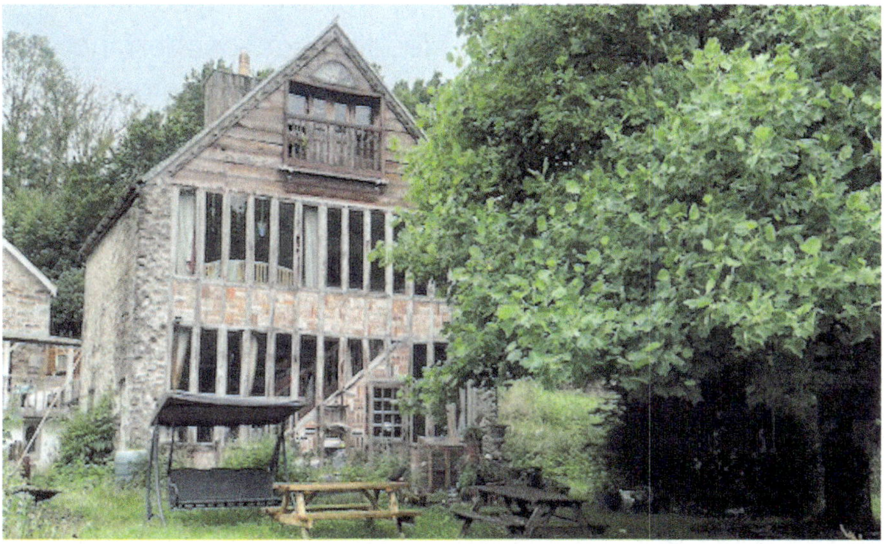

Here in my new home, which I named my healing sanctuary, I went deep into healing. I learnt trauma release exercises, meditating, journeying, reiki, doing yoga, sitting on the earth, taking long walks in nature. All of these were practices I had used daily before having Dorothy. I had always been told as a child I was 'sensitive' and as an adult that I was 'too sensitive'. I always followed my intuition, listened to my Earth Mother for guidance, communed with guides and angels, and followed my inner cyclic seasons as a spiritual practice. I had a large medicine bag with plenty of tools that I knew would support me. My body was recovering from the trauma of community life, but some symptoms stayed. In particular the mid cycle bleeding was concerning me. I could feel what I thought were polyps on my cervix, pain with my moon time. I was to and fro from the doctors for five months before they finally agreed to a scan and an appointment with a gynaecologist.

The scan was all clear (I was convinced it was going to show fibroids- but no). However the gynae appointment was another story. I was examined by inserting a camera so they could get a large image of my cervix up on the screen I was shocked by what I saw and I could tell by the faces of the nurse and doctor that it wasn't looking good. Very quickly they did a biopsy. I'm not even sure I was aware what they were doing, as it's not something I'd have agreed to and would probably have refused if I'd had time to process what was happening in that moment. I was then bundled out of the examination room being told I'd hear the results in about a week.

Then I did what you should never do - I looked at 'Dr Google'!! Oh, there are some scary pictures, diagrams and photos on line, and while one part of me was working hard to convince me it would all be fine, another was screaming it was cervical cancer!

The results came in quickly. Which made me think this wasn't going to be good news, especially as only a couple of days had passed since my appointment, and they insisted I went in to see the doctor to get the results face to face.

A friend came with me, I recommend *always taking a friend,* as sometimes it's hard to take in all the information, and having another person who isn't so emotionally involved means that they can take notes and ask the questions you may not have considered. A bit like a cancer doula! We sat in a little office to get the results. I found out I had a rare kind of cancer (one that's not detected by smears). It was early (stage 1b), and I would be passed along to the oncology gynaecology department. I was given some leaflets about cervical cancer and sent on my way.

That's the practical bit. But here's what was going on inside me as soon as I heard 'It's cancer' I felt an energy shift. Something inside me went "it's fine, I know what to do". A calmness descended on me. Even the doctor noticed as she asked if I was okay and if I needed a sweet tea and a biscuit, (yes, they offer people with cancer sugary snacks!). As we left, both my friend and I commented on how the energy in the room changed and how we had felt a presence - an angel in the room?! (remember this bit as there's more to this later).

I was blessed that, on the same day, at roughly the same time, my friend Sally was having her oncologist appointment upstairs from me, and when I walked out of the hospital there she was, smiling and waiting for me. I blurted out 'it's cancer' and she responded in her Scottish accent "och, it'll be fine, just get it cut out and then it's over!" To which I replied "no way are they cutting out my womb!" I think we were both surprised at each others reactions- Sally had taken the surgery route when she had been first diagnosed, but with the secondary cancer she was on a natural healing journey. All three of us headed to the nearest M&S cafe for a cuppa and to get over the shock. None of us could face going back to the 'real world' just yet.

Looking back, it's so surreal to think about getting a cancer diagnosis and within seconds your whole life is changed. Everything looks the same, people around you are getting on with life, but your life has just been turned on its head and no one knows.

I can't even remember what we talked about in that cafe, but I imagine it was probably a discussion about what my next steps might be.

I do remember my friend and I driving back to pick up the children, who were staying with another friend, and Tom being there waiting for me and just bursting into tears and saying it's cancer as he held me. I didn't want to speak to my friend who had the children, I just wanted to go home and go back to 'normal'.

Initially we decided not to tell the children, who at this point they were eight and six years old. However I did tell the 2 older ones immediately and joked that there was nothing to worry about; I was a womb whisperer and would be fine! I had an idea that the cancer was small and would be easily cleared. But within a few weeks of starting full on protocols of diet changes, liver packs, and enemas, it was clear to the children something was going on. I called Macmillan for advice on how to talk to the children without scaring them, and they suggested some great books (see the resources section), which we read together, although most of the books do have bits about 'mummy or daddy going to hospital/having treatment'- which I repeatedly said I wouldn't be doing, as I knew out bodies can heal without that!. I was, and have been all the way through my healing, totally in awe of the resilience of my children. Dorothy was pretty open about it with her friends and at school, but didn't milk it and use it to get pity. Emrys is more quiet and sensitive and had his own ways of dealing with it. He talked to me a lot and prayed for my healing whenever we visited sacred places, or did any ritual or ceremony- he never asked for anything for himself, he always sent love out to others and especially Mummy.

Then came the appointment with the doctor representing the oncology gynae team. To this day I still struggle with the knowledge that a whole team can meet to discuss and make big life changing decisions about your case without you present! Anyway, they had decided it would be best for me to have a radical hysterectomy- ermmm NO! After years of womb work they want to chop out my sacred womb? No, no, no. I even went so far as to ask the doctor (a man of course) if he had a tiny bit of cancer on the end of his penis- would he chop it off? He didn't reply! I pretty much walked out of that meeting refusing their care and with a strong inner knowing I could heal.

I was really curious about my cervix diagnosis, and found it fascinating that I'd been holding women's circles, working as a doula, supporting women with their fertility for almost thirty years. All that time I'd been doing what I called 'womb work' but I hadn't really considered the cervix, apart from when I was in labour willing it to open. So this was my first pull for my healing, to my cervix, I began a daily dialogue with her and she was pretty put out that she'd been ignored and not included in my work. I took a deep dive into the mysteries of the cervix and met her in the place of mystical portal that she truly is. I also decided to blog about this deep journey, just incase it was helpful to others with cervical issues or for anyone who wanted to go deeper into the mysteries of the womb, our cycles and the cervix! I sat with what to name it and the obvious hit me: Hello Cervix! This was literally the greeting to my holy body each day. www.hellocervix.me.uk

I also had an 'awakening' around love at this time.

I was cleaning my son's room a few days after being given the 'C' word and I just got flooded with emotion. I suppose it was being surrounded by his toys, looking at his pictures on the wall and wondering how all this might affect him, I felt completely overwhelmed with sadness for my children as well as myself I remember sitting on the floor, crying, the sunlight on my face and screaming inside "why me, what about my children, why is this happening?" And a really clear voice came through "LET THE LOVE IN". I cried even more then, realising how shut down I had become from the trauma of leaving the community and leaving Tom. I had gone into survival mode and was in that "I can do it MYSELF" mode . This was one in which I'd spent most of my life, having been a single mum with my eldest children from the age of nineteen onwards. It was time to soften, to open my heart and let in the help. I sat there for quite a while, with my tears, the sun (which felt like a healing presence) and a gradual peeling away of the heart amour I had put around myself, I stepped out of that room feeling so much lighter on all levels!

I hadn't told many people about the diagnosis, just close family. But this opening to love moved me to start a social media group called 'Let the Love in' I added people I knew would be supportive and asked them to send me positive quotes, memes, messages of support. This soon became a place I could reach out for help. Towards the end of my healing I even opened it up to others who had cancer so we could share the love even more.

I was blogging my journey, which was both cathartic for me and hopefully helpful for others, as well as being another way of keeping friends and family in the loop of what was happening. I set up a 'Patreon' so people could support me financially, and which I also called 'Let the Love in'. I would post updates and little tools and practices I was using in exchange for their monthly donations.

This support was truly amazing, I even had people I'd never met joining my Patreon! It was a creation of community, of new bonding friendships and a deepening of old friendships.

The next eighteen months was a process of intensive self-healing. This included appointments with naturopath/nutritionist, herbalist and acupuncturist as well as going for hyperbaric oxygen, doing daily yoga, breath work, yoni steams, nature connection (putting my yoni on the Earth most days!), meditation, drinking lots of water and green juices, eating alkaline foods, daily liver packs and enemas, fasting, taking numerous supplements and awful tasting concoctions!

Looking back, I can see that what I didn't do enough of was changing my behaviours. I was still working too much, stressed with the daily routines (adding in more to those with the healing practices, while not letting go of some of what I was already doing), I had very little money and I hardly asked for help. I can see now that I had too much of an 'I can do this myself' attitude, even though I had the support of my groups and friends. I also hadn't faced my mortality. I hadn't really faced death, and I hadn't fully chosen life! Read more on that later.

Stepping away from the allopathic system, I was out on my own, with no one checking if what I was doing was working. Everyone was telling me I looked great, and I was hoping that looking great on the outside meant I was healing inside, but I didn't know for sure, there was a constant lurking thought of "what if it's not working?"

So I went back to the gynaecologist feeling empowered and knowing what I wanted, I reminded myself 'these doctors are here to support me- they do what I want' and first and foremost I asked for a female doctor to work with, which they agreed to. I then began having three monthly internal checks and a scan every six months or so (when I requested). They were happy for me to do my own thing and 'assured' me there was always the option of surgery. My sense was that they saw me as a bit of a wacko and maybe an interesting experiment for them to observe!

I also wrote to the practice manager of my GP surgery and requested to be able to have blood tests whenever I wanted without having to see my GP first, as had previously been the case, and they agreed. This is taking your health into your own hands! I would even ask to insert the speculum myself when I had internals.

After around fifteen months of intensive healing protocols I had an internal exam where the gynaecologist said if I had just come to her, she would say my cervix was totally healthy. She suggested we use the machine with a camera so she could have a good look around, and even take photos. Everything looked clear! I was over joyed, I had cleared this rare cancer, staged at 1b within eighteen months! I also knew not to get too complacent, as I had known someone to have an all clear and within a few months have it return.

So I kept up my healthy eating regime, protocols, supplements and carried on with life.

Back to work, back to stress, mothering, relationships. By this time Tom and I had got back together- well a cancer diagnosis makes you look at what's really important in life. It wasn't easy but we were working on things and having counselling.

Once again I had less time, (or maybe I wasn't making enough time?) for self nourishment.

The truth was I hadn't made enough changes to really shift my life!

Fast forward four months, and I'm supporting a friend who has lost her partner in a tragic accident. I'm out in Portugal and of course, she's in massive grief. With another friend we are sorting the practical things, like scooping up her children, making food, cleaning and tidying. At the same time we are holding sacred space for the grief process, doing little rituals, going to the beach to make offerings, feeling into the beauty of death while holding the massive waves of emotion my friend was going through.

I'm balancing it with my self-care, so eating well, spending time on the earth, meditating, and making the most of being somewhere beautiful and warm. But it's hard, it's beautiful, it's painful to witness the loss of a beloved. There are amazing synchronicities happening for all of us, helping us feel that this is all part of the divine plan, while my friend falls deep into the despair of loss. It was such an honour to witness someone in the full ecstasy of grief, the highs and the deep lows. It was a huge lesson in just holding space, that you can't make anything better, all you can do is be there, loving them.

We come home and the wider community catch my friend with open arms, cooking for her and her children, supporting where they can, while giving her space to grieve.

But it's March 2020, the first stirrings of 'covid' are happening, and the world is about to change for everyone and especially me!

I'm having slight pain on my right side. I'm wondering if its my appendix, but decide to wait and see if it gets worse before having to deal with seeing a doctor while it's all masks and spacesuits in there because of the pandemic. After a week or so I'm realising it's not getting any better, so I manage to get an appointment at my GP surgery (not easy at that time!) and she examines me, looks at my notes and then assures me it's probably one of my ovarian cysts. "What ovarian cysts?" I ask. "Oh your last scan showed cysts on your ovaries, we should probably do another scan to check." So she books me in for an MRI, but who knows how long that might be, and tells me to go to A&E if the pain worsens.

So I go home and start reading my womb books on what to do to support ovarian cysts; I start to add herbs, womb massage and castor oil packs on my ovaries to my routine. But the pain is getting worse and I can feel my ovaries growing day by day.

I go to A&E, which, lucky for me, is unusually quiet, due to the ward and department closures as a result of covid. I'm seen quickly and get sent up to the gynae ward, where coincidentally the doctor who first diagnosed me is on duty. Bearing in mind it's been almost two years since I saw her- she remembers me and asks "why didn't you get the hysterectomy?"

I'm not really in the mood to go into this and brush her off saying "well, I wanted to do natural healing, rather than surgery." She examines me and sends me for a ultrasound scan to see what's going on. I always find it weird that the only ultra sound machines I have seen are in the maternity unit. Today it's empty in here, but other times I've had to have a scan, it's felt strange sitting with pregnant mothers when I could potentially being told I could never have children again. To be fair, I don't want any more, but it made me think of younger women in my position and how insensitive this feels.

I have my scan and can see clearly on the screen my ovaries are huge, distorted and way higher up in my body than usual. I can also see there's loads of fluid all around my pelvis and abdomen and sense this is more serious than cysts.

Back to the doctors room, where she wants to refer me for a biopsy. I refuse, as I know that biopsies can cause cancer to spread (if it is cancer? I still have hope it could just be cysts gone wild?) I tell her I want another opinion.

All the way along the journey dealing with doctors, I had to stay so strong in my convictions. Yes there are times when compromise is necessary, but know your own body, know your truth, and know what feels okay for you and what doesn't.

I'm now referred to a gynea oncologist in Swansea (over an hour away) and begin to surrender to the hysterectomy route.

Eventually, after waiting for MRI and PET scans plus another scan that left me radioactive for twelve *hours*(!) which meant not being around my children for twelve hours- goddess knows that that did to my body!!!! I finally get an appointment with the gynea oncologist after weeks of waiting.

Top Tip- high doses of elemental magnesium and DMSO taken three days before scans help protect the body from harm. I also took loads of spirulina, coriander and seaweeds in a smoothie afterwards which have heavy metals removing properties.

Each time I get an appointment with a new doctor I send love ahead of me, I ask my guides for the very best person to work with me and let go, trusting that all will be well.

We drive to Swansea - remember it's covid times, so I have to go in to the appointment alone. The doctors are all masked up and the first thing one of them says looking up from my notes is, "Why didn't you have the hysterectomy in 2018?" This is neither helpful, nor a good start. I try to stay humble and put myself in their hands. There are two doctors in the room- one male, one female along with a nurse, and it feels somewhat over crowded. They read through the scan results: huge masses on the ovaries and a mass of around 8cm in the womb- probably cancer that spread from the cervix (without a biopsy there's no way to know for sure- but it's very likely these masses are cancer). They ask to do an internal examination, both vaginal and anal (I'm glad I did an enema before this appointment!) along with an external exam of my abdomen. As if having one exam isn't enough, the second doctor goes in for another opinion. They report back that the masses feel hard, indicating cancer, and the ligaments around my womb also feel hard and therefore it's likely the cancer has spread. This means it's too late for a hysterectomy and the only treatment they can offer is chemo/ radiotherapy.

I stumble out. Tom and the children are waiting in the car, I shake my head, "it's not good". I sit and sob all the way home- emotions flitting from rage to self pity.

I’m in shock, inside I'm screaming ‘NOOOOOOO’.

The words ‘too late’ are going around and around in my head. My thoughts are spinning. “How did this happen? How can it be too late? Why did I leave it too late? But I just surrendered to a hysterectomy...and now I have to change my mind again? I don't want chemo/radio!! What am I going to do?”

And then to blame... “The other consultant should have flagged up these 'cysts' she saw on my scan. Why did she say everything was okay? Why didn't she insist on keeping a check on me? Why didn't she suggest more scans?”

My brain is trying somehow to make everything okay.

But it's not okay. The seriousness of the situation just stepped up: so I have to step up to meet it. It's time to try things I haven't tried, and up my game. More castor oil packs, more enemas, more green juice, more water, more supplements, more research. Looking into urine therapy, getting in touch with a doctor for mistletoe and booking an appointment with a Cannabis Clinic. Fundraising to help pay for private treatment, an oxygen machine for at home (the hyperbaric oxygen place closed due to covid!) plus a second opinion (thank you Team Verrico who paid for that).

I'm talking to my womb and ovaries, and massaging DMSO and frankincense into my abdomen, whilst trying not to freak out, as I can feel the growths getting bigger by the day.

Loving my body, meditating on being radiant and vibrant, visualising my future self, whole and well has become my main focus.

And time is on my side, because of this 'pandemic' we are in, nothing happens fast and I feel blessed that the more time I have before the wheels of 'treatment' start, the more time I have to work on my healing.

I wake up in pain – this is serious, mega pain in my abdomen. I feel like I'm dying. I can't move, I'm curled up in a ball, sweating from the pain, delirious from the pain. Tom calls A&E, we all bundle into the car, to this day I have no idea how Tom got me clothed and out into the car.

Friends meet us on route and take the kids- I remember their scared faces "is mummy going to be okay?" "I'll be okay", I whisper. We get to A&E where Tom bundles me into a wheelchair and tells the porter what's happened.

He's told he's not allowed in and goes off to the bench opposite the hospital to wait. I'm almost fainting with pain and then have to give the receptionist my details. I remember feeling so dizzy and sweating loads, just wondering what the hell is going on with my body.

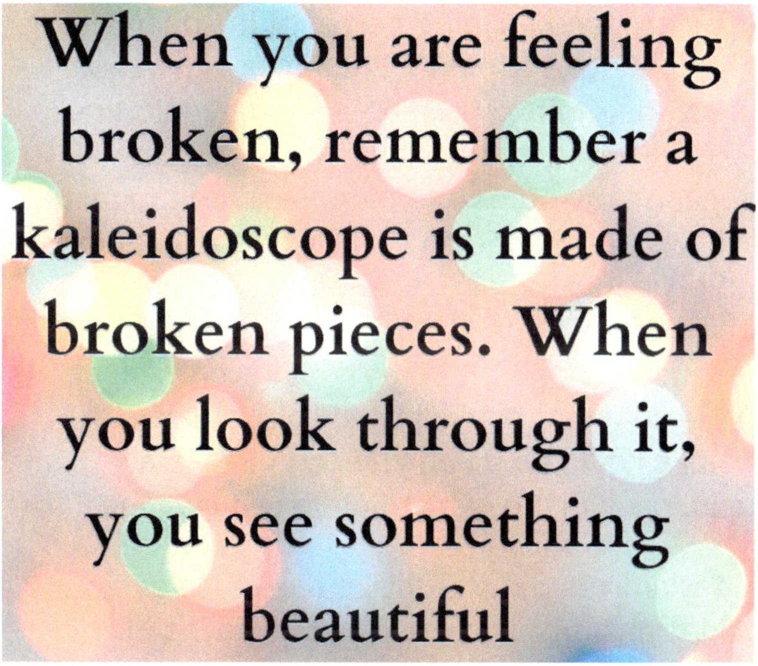

I'm taken to a room with a bed, where they do blood pressure, take my temperature, all the 'usual' tests and am told it's busy and I'll have to wait for a doctor. I'm literally there for hours, I think at one point I was offered tea and a sandwich, but don't see a doctor. A nurse pops in now and again to check on me. The pain is lessening, I keep asking if I'm going to have a scan or anything, but no one knows. I'm texting Tom to let him know, and he keeps phoning the A&E for updates and to put a bit of pressure on.

Hours later a doctor comes in and says they have spoken to my oncologist and made an appointment for me to see her tomorrow morning at 9.30am, and I can go home; "if the pain continues, take aspirin". I'm fuming! I've been here all day, in excruciating pain to be told this? Reading between the lines, I think they saw cancer on my notes and didn't want to touch me. Plus, we are now going to have to get up at 6am and drive to Swansea for another doctors appointment! So it's back home, dosed up on pain meds and I have a really bad night's sleep on the sofa bed downstairs (I can't make it upstairs I'm in so much pain) and then start again, back in the car and off to see my Onc.

She examines me and thinks one of my cysts or ovaries has ruptured, which explains the intense pain and why it's now easing. She says she will discuss urgent surgery with her team. This definitely means removal of the ovaries, possibly the womb as well, depending what they find once they open me up. I will still have to have the chemo/radio after surgery. They will have a team meeting and let me know.

Part of me feels relieved. Surgery I can cope with, although I'm still unsure about the other treatments. But I remind myself 'lets do this a step at a time'. Plus I feel this change in 'plans' once more gives me a bit of breathing space to get my head around what's going to happen next and focus on getting strong and well. I wonder if this 'rupture' has been a blessing in disguise?

I’m still focussed on getting a second opinion. I had requested one a while ago, they aren't cheap and I was getting support from the charity Team Verrico, so it was all being organised through them. The doctor I spoke with seemed very knowledgeable and all, however he was still an allopathic doctor who pretty much agreed with the treatment plan my own doctor had come up with. I was disappointed, as I was hoping to find a doctor who might support something like intravenous vitamin C and mistletoe, but it seems such doctors don’t exist in the UK.

After several phone calls with my oncologist, and one where I had to insist my lymph nodes weren't removed during surgery, a date was organised for July 2020. It had been five months since my first appointment with my GP about abdominal pain.

As part of my coming to terms with surgery, losing my ovaries, maybe my womb, I called together my women friends, in order to be heard, to be witnessed and to be painted. As I lay in the middle of a circle of these beautiful women, who had held me and cared for my children, (I had such gratitude for my community and my friends) they sang to me, painted my swollen cancer full belly with henna- painting healing symbols, whispering words of encouragement and love.

Literally days before my surgery, it gets postponed. Oh my, how many more times can I surrender and trust? Over and over it seems!

Again this feels a blessing – another date is set – and a few days before I have a bleed, my last ever moon blood. How many women get to know that this one is the last? Once more I call in some friends. I want to be reborn in the river. I've had a bit of an obsession the past few months with baptism, not in the church sense, but in the 'washing away, being cleansed by our Earth Mother'. This feels like the time!

Friends come and we walk to the river below my house. We smudge, drum, and sing. I get naked and they paint my whole body with ochre. Then I wade into the river, offering myself, ochre, moon blood and all, to the waters, to Mother Earth, thanking them for their holding and support, asking to be washed clean; to be born again, whole, radiant and perfect! I dunk under (it's FREEZING!!). I'm screaming from the cold and pretty quickly climb out feeling renewed. We sit by the river a while before heading home for a hot cuppa.

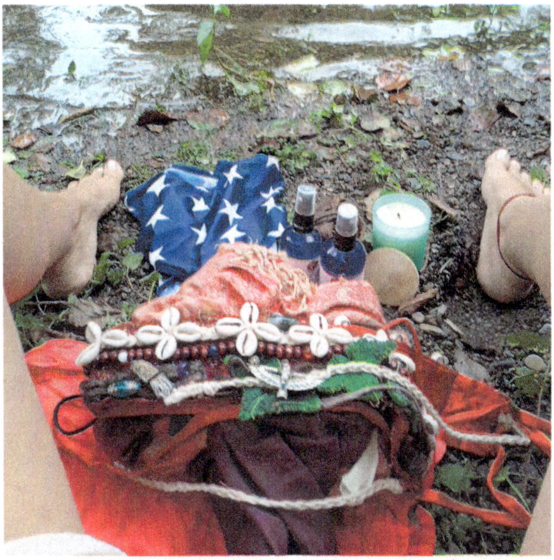

Now I'm ready for whatever they are going to do in that hospital. I'm ready. I've had a Brandon Bay Journey with a friend, and flower essence consultation so I've got my perfect medicine to hand, and I've faced all my fears, let go of everything I need to let go of. Bring it on!

I get to the hospital the afternoon before the op is scheduled, apparently at 8.30am the next morning, so I'll be first on the table, which I think is good as those surgeons will be fresh at the start of the day! It's all very surreal. Of course I'm nervous, doing my breathing exercises in the car on the way there. Tom is allowed to carry my bags up but not allowed on the ward. We have an emotional goodbye. It's all very weird.

I've got a bag full of juices, smoothies, fresh fruit, snacks and treats as I know what the hospital food will be like! Along with Rescue Remedy, personal remedy blends from friends, homeopathic remedies, supplements, all things to aid healing! Plus crystals, a medicine pouch with power items from my women friends, oracle cards, loads of books, my tablet to watch movies, my iPod with soothing music and meditations....I'm surrounded by my healing stuff!

I'm also adorning my F*!k Cancer t-shirt!

There are various tests to be done, bloods to be taken, apparently some pre-op meds sometime in the night. There are a couple of other women on the ward, although it sounds as if they are due to be discharged pretty soon. Everyone is friendly and nice (despite the masks!). The TV is on in the corner, but I turn away and read one of my books.

I don't sleep well. The ward has dim lights on all night and I'm woken for tests and meds. But it seems the meds were given too late, so surgery will be later in the day. More surrender.

I can't help but listen to a woman talking to her surgeon behind the curtain opposite me. She has a lump in her neck, and the surgeon sounds confident it will be a simple op and that the cancer hasn't spread. He actually sounds very cocky and I'm glad my surgeon is a woman!

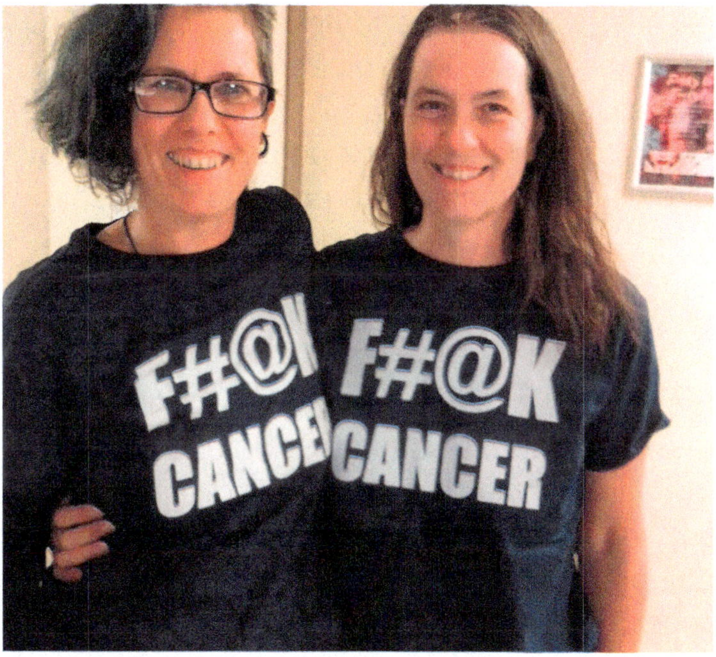

(Although my anaesthetist who talks me through the anaesthetic options for my surgery seems to have a huge ego -and huge mask!)

Anyway, my doctor comes to talk me through the surgery, and just drops in "and if we find that cancer has spread to the bowel, do you give permission for us to remove it?" I'm like...WTAF? "It's just before surgery and now you're talking about bowel removal, what does that even mean? Why hasn't this been mentioned before?"

"Well, it's just in case, and if we do need to remove the bowel, it will mean having a stoma." "A stoma, what's a stoma? A poo bag? You're seriously asking me to give permission to remove my bowel and fit me with a poo bag? Now?"

Again, SURRENDER. "OKAY, fine, do whatever it takes."

I sign the papers, truly feeling I'm signing my life away. I'm put into a surgical gown and wheeled away, although not before texting my 'healing group' of friends who are all gonna sing, chant, drum, pray, send reiki ...all of it with bells on. Alongside my shamanic friends who I have asked to keep my soul tethered, as I don't wanna be flying off while I'm under the knife! Now I'm start ing to feel the 'this is it' excitement/anxiety sensation. It's so strange because no one wants to be cut open; no one wants to go through such an ordeal. Besides, from studying trauma, we know that we 'disengage' from the body when it goes through trauma, and I know this will be traumatic. Yet somehow I begin to feel calm, peaceful even.

The surgery feels full and busy. A nice nurse squeezes my hand and asks if I'm okay. I nod, I'm fine I tell her (she doesn't look like she believes me!). Then before I know it the anaesthetic is going in. I sense my dad with me and the next thing I remember is waking up and saying "What did you take?".

The nurse and surgeon look shocked, "I've never seen someone come around so alert! We removed your ovaries, drained about 2 litres of fluid. We did some exploratory examinations but couldn't remove the womb, the ligaments were too hardened." I burst into tears (part relief- I still have my womb! Part disappointment as I know now that chemo/radio will be the next suggestion). "What about the bowel?" I ask, "Your bowel looked fine". Well that's something!

I'm wheeled back to the ward, which is empty, and have a little peek under my gown. I was shaved (they didn't mention they would do that!), I have a catheter in (they said that would happen), and I have a huge covering from the bottom of my ribs down to my pubic bone. I was kinda expecting something a bit smaller. I guess the wound underneath might be smaller than the medical gauze?

I make a little video on my phone letting family and friends know I'm okay and lie down to listen to some healing music and have a snooze. I'm a bit in a daze (probably from the drugs!) but also just feeling how surreal all of this is.

I'm woken to have my blood pressure checked, and temp taken. They check on my pain and administer some more medication. I ask about the woman who was in the bed opposite me. I had felt for her as her story sounded like such a fast cancer diagnosis to surgery I thought maybe I could offer her a bit of support.

Just to note, this is what the medical profession do. As soon as they find cancer it's on with the treatment ASAP, before you have time to process what's going on. I always advise folk to take their time on deciding treatment; after all it's your body, not theirs! Shockingly I'm told that her surgery took nine hours and she ended up having a double mastectomy due to the cancer having spread much further than they thought. So she'd been put in a room on her own as it's so much for her to deal with. Oh my, the poor woman, and after I had thought how cocky her surgeon sounded.

I suddenly feel so grateful for my 'small' op, and how thorough my surgeon had been, so I knew exactly what to expect. Something inside me stirs. A deep knowing that I need to take the chemotherapy, and I need to transmute it into golden, healing light and I need to heal my womb. I contemplate my journey from the start when I refused the hysterectomy. I was adamant I would keep my womb and gosh, what a miracle I still have her- but what is she now?

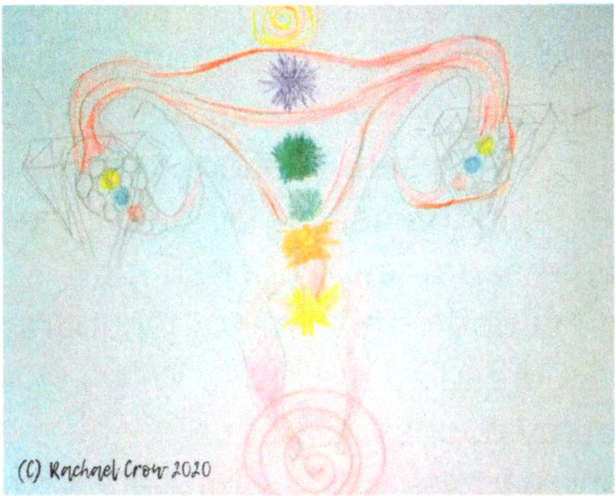

"I am your sacred inner altar" comes the reply. Wow.

I have a couple of days recuperating and pretty much as soon as the catheter is out and my bladder and bowels are working okay, and I can walk to the bathroom by myself, I'm allowed to go home. I'm packed up into a wheelchair with a bag full of drugs, including loads of pain relief meds and blood thinners to self- inject. Tom comes to pick me up. I'm wheeled to the car and struggle to get in the front seat. I'm realising how my abdominal muscles are used for ALL movement!!

I'm so happy to be home, and to have my children with me. Friends are popping by most days with nourishing meals, juices and smoothies (and for Tom and the kids!), plus little gifts of love. Some stay and have a chat, some just drop off and go. I'm grateful for it all.

The weather is glorious and as soon as I feel okay going up and down stairs, I'm out in the garden on the swing seat, resting and soaking up the sun, breathing the healing air under the trees. Or lying on the earth, feeling her support underneath my body. This time of recuperation is the part I was dreading the most. When I had spoken with my counsellor about having the operation she had asked me whether I worried about it, and I'd answered, "I don't think I can do nothing for six weeks and I don't think Tom can run the house on his own!" She repeated that back to me and asked if those were my biggest worries over having surgery?! It all seems ridiculous now, as actually resting is easy when your body restricts you from too much movement and Tom was doing just fine. It was a lesson in both letting go and allowing people to step up for you. It's always good for others (and ourselves) to really witness how many responsibilities we hold when we let go of them.

There was also an anticipation hovering over us as we waited for the biopsy results. I just kept pushing it out of my mind, telling myself 'no news is good news'. Although we were all pretty sure it was cancer, I hadn't considered if it was that, it would be classed as secondary cancer and the impact that might have on me, and the treatment plan they would offer.

Finally 'the call' came, after waiting five weeks since the operation. I had one ovary with metastasised cervical cancer. It had spread. Yep guessed that already. We knew there was spread to the womb and ligaments, and there was concern that it would be in the lymph now too, so they want to throw a pretty high dose of chemo and radiotherapy at me to prevent any more spread. I'm restaged at stage 4 …oh the labels. I quickly decided to stay positive. After all, I'm the same person I was yesterday whatever label / stage they want to give me…..

…..so I'm not taking on their numbers or stages and I will continue to live life!

I keep trusting in the divine plan and following my intuition, working on bringing the positivity back in. Whatever life keeps throwing at me, I will keep rising!

It was being re-staged that was the shock. I soooo wasn't expecting that. I understand that they are covering themselves, saying there's no guarantee treatment will work, all we can offer you is palliative care…But hey, there's no guarantees in life are there?

Every day I have swinging emotions, at times, almost laughing at what life keeps giving me … really…more? Wow you must think I'm superhuman to keep throwing all this at me? And then going into 'why me… I can't handle this'. But I recognise this pattern as what I go through every time life throws me a curve ball, and the process through it gets faster and faster each time. So I stick with being gentle with myself, allowing it all to flow through, staying grounded, and in touch with loving friends and family. I continue to feel all the love and support all around me and not wallow too long in the 'why me' bit!

Although that bit is important to really feel into; feel the grief, feel the little scared girl inside. Feel the anger/rage and let it flow through. I have a three day rule- no wallowing past three days!

Although I do feel like I'm living about five lifetimes worth of lessons crammed into this one life!

As a friend said- stage 4 is the club no one wants to join- but I will say, I've met some amazing, inspirational stage 4 thrivers in this club!

My mum always said to me that none of us are perfect and there are always lessons to learn, always more ways to grow. It never ends. That's why we have chosen to incarnate here on earth, to experience life as a human with all it's ups and downs. I'm certainly experiencing life as I never imagined! If we're still alive, there's still more to do/be/learn! And in these time, anything is possible. So I choose to put my energy into creating the best possible life.

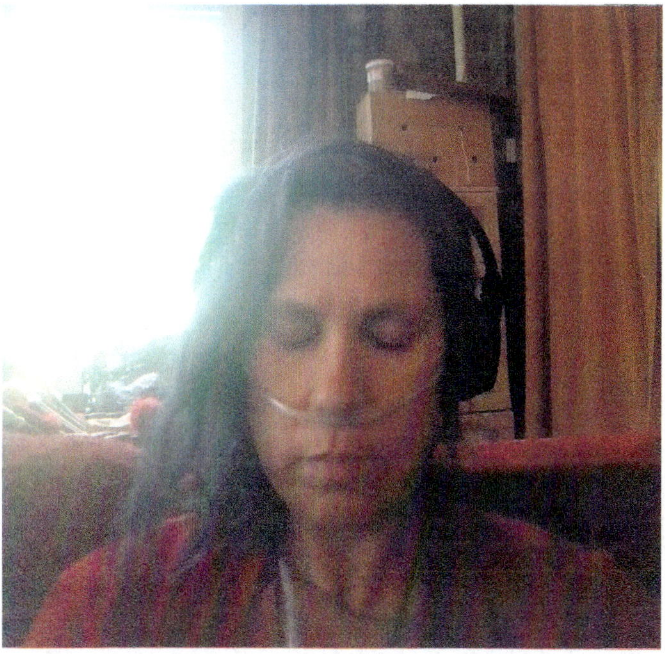

So, whats next? I have an appointment to see the seeing the chemo/radiologist. I have begun mistletoe injections and will hopefully fit in going to the clinic in Stroud and have IV drip of mistletoe treatment soon, plus all my usual protocol of juicing, liver packs, enemas, meditations, healing etc.

I've got my eye on a week long Joe Dispenza retreat in London which could be life changing, and I plan a head shaving fundraiser for the charity Team Vericco who have supported me weekly by paying for my counselling and for organic veg. My head will be shaved on a Facebook live video which feels exciting and positive. Challenging how I feel about my looks, and my hair!

I continue to share my story on my blog and social media, breaking the cancer taboos, staying positive, healing, and living life to the FULL with LOVE & JOY! And hopefully helping and inspiring others.

My inner healing continues. I'm following Dr Joe Dispenza's online progressive workshop and have just completed a forty day Course in Miracles group journey– focussing on my divinity over any dis-ease.

I have a surprise from my friends -a gift of a woollen blanket- decorated with the words 'I did it my way', plus lots of hearts, fabric flowers, beads, trinkets. I was completely overwhelmed by its arrival …my amazing community gathered to create this for me (and those further away posted bits to be added) so I can be wrapped in their love. It seems to be a new tradition as earlier this year I was part of a group making a butterfly blanket for another of our red tent sisters. It just shows how our women's groups really do create a lasting community. We haven't gathered in circle for a long time but the holding energy is still strong. I feel so blessed to have such special friends.

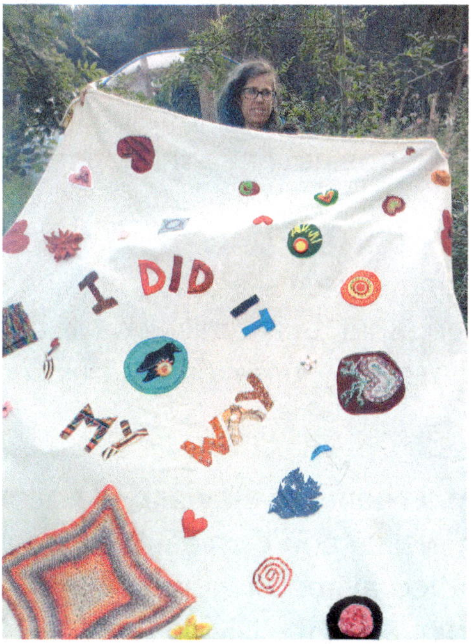

All through my healing journey I have said I will 'Do It My Way' and even though I'm now following more of the allopathic route, I am doing it my way! Which includes fasting to support my healthy cells while I undergo chemotherapy- as recommended by the book The Longevity Diet and under the guidance of my various natural healing team members.

Fasting creates a ‘magic shield’ around the healthy cells and leaves the sick cells hungry, so they suck up the chemo (which was due to start on the 23rd Sept). I’m also using Mistletoe Therapy to support the wellness of my immune system, along with all the other protocols of enemas, liver packs, and an organic diet.

I am no longer using the C word in reference to myself, Instead, I am affirming health. I am a radiant, vibrant being. I’m connecting with my energy body and love, love, love.

I’m prioritising self-care and my healing over work, trusting that as a family we will be held- on all levels; financially, emotionally, physically, and spiritually.

My eldest son came to stay and we had days on the beach, walks, and picnics. We also visited St Davids Cathedral and St Nons chapel with such beautiful images of the Divine feminine, Mother Mary and St Non. I had visited here two years before and so much had changed in my life since then. I felt very emotional sitting in the chapel, thinking over the years and my gratitude for my deepening relationship with Our Lady, Beloved Mary.

The head shaving fundraiser is a success, and I'm even joined by my husband and two other friends from Bristol. Together we raise over £500 for Team Vericco and a few hundred for my personal fundraiser. I shave my head live on my Facebook page and share the video on my blog. Luckily, I don't look too bad with a shaved head!

Memories of a past life as a Buddhist nun begins to filter though- another layer of my inner healing.

Chemo starts, I follow my inner guidance with all the treatments I've using. What came up with chemo was to see it as love, liquid love, love elixir flowing into my body, healing and supporting my body to let go of the cancer cells.

Love heals. Love is all there is. Tune into Love. Be love. You are Held.

These are the messages coming in to my life- so I choose to trust these messages!

Sitting in the hospital (lovely comfy chairs, kind nurses- six hours to myself to meditate and tune into love) I imagined myself totally wrapped in light. Mother Mary and Yeshua came in and I feel them beaming loving, healing light into the drip. I see healing light flowing though my veins. All day I just sit in light and love. I have received so many messages from family and friends that have topped me up and supported me in feeling completely held.

On arriving home I rest, have a lovely long soak in the bath. Time to up the self care even more.

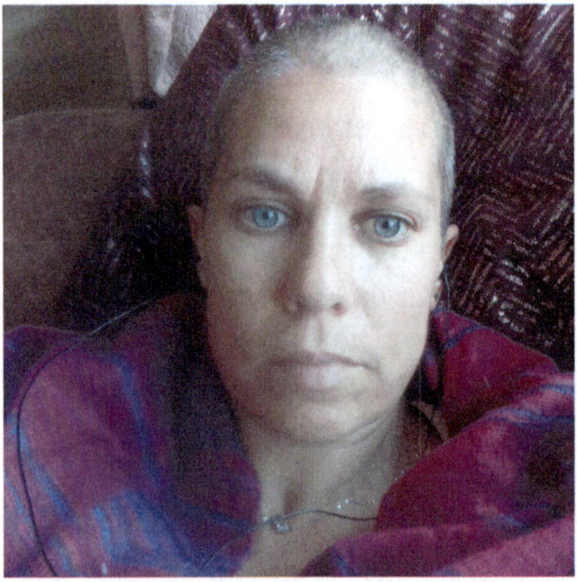

The days after the chemo I rest. I have slight nausea, so I drink ginger and mint tea, plenty of water, take slippery elm, aloe vera and magnesium citrate to support my digestion, and eat small, light meals. The sensations in my achy body progress through-out the day until by evening my womb has intense pain (liver and womb packs and hot water bottles are such a comfort!). I go to bed listening to a meditation but wake all through the night aching and having hot flushes.

Each time I caught myself sinking into 'pain' I replaced the thought with

"I am an Infinite Being, I am not subject to that" from Healing and Recovery by David Hawkins

I choose to connect in with my light, energy body over my 3D body.

I am Radiant, I am Vibrant, I am Whole.

I rest and stay in the vibration of love and gratitude- despite being still achy and suffering nausea! I am constantly upping my self care. I walk barefoot outside to support detoxing, I sip herb teas, listening to Dr Joe meditations and watching his talks, following my body's guidance.

I'm also totally open to receiving healing, prayers … all modalities from anyone who offers! Beam me up!

I travel to Stroud for my first lot of IV Mistletoe, I'm also hoping to soon start IV vitamin C. The treatments need to be spaced out to get the best results between chemo rounds.

Mistletoe is something I highly recommend! It's not for all cancers so do some research, I have links on my healing blog where you can contact doctors who will prescribe and administer it. I felt AMAZING on mistletoe.

I'm blessed to have my dear friend Dominique near the doctors where I have the IV mistletoe, so after my first round I'm tucked up on her sofa, and she's giving me a cranial treatment (how lucky am I?), while my body takes in this ancient medicine. The doctor had explained that IV vitamin C needs to be taken at least a week away from mistletoe so thats not on the cards for me at the moment, as it would be way too much travelling.

This becomes part of my new routine. Mistletoe between rounds of chemo, a beautiful friend from my 'old life' in Bristol offers to meet me on the motorway and drive me to Stroud. Louise knows Dominique so we have 'girls night' which makes these visits extra special.

The day before my next round of chemo I have a swim at a local beach with two girl friends, in honour of my Cancer Sistar Sally, who sadly never made it for a cold swim after us both saying we would give it a go for the last year or so! So I have decided to keep it up for myself and in Sally's name. It's a beautiful sunny morning, the water is freezing cold, so there's much swearing and shouting to help me ease into the water. Following my acupuncturists instructions, I don't stay in for too long, but I do feel SO INVIGORATED afterwards and am very happy to crack open my hot flask of herbal tea in the sun and relax on the beach afterwards, fully dressed of course!

Then my next chemo session. This time I'm listening to the Chemotherapy Companion from Hemi Synch, visualising chemo as a love potion, created with love… especially for me.

Chemo as love medicine.

With each drop going into my body I'm imagining drips of LOVE, LOVE, LOVE…

Arriving home from hospital I begin to prepare for my Dark moon offering. Earlier in the week (on my birthday to be exact!) I was able to go back to Swansea and collect my ovaries, since I had arranged for them to be kept for me after the hospital had finished biopsying them. Because of my surgery recovery and then starting chemo, collection hadn't been easy to arrange. But I seized the opportunity and got my Birthday Ovaries! How many people can say they got ovaries for their birthday? (I also went to the fabulous V Hub for lunch and went wig shopping!).

That evening, after my wonderful hubby had dug a hole under my rose bush, I cleansed myself with home grown sage. I then made prayers and began with offerings of my hair I had shaved off, cotton moon pads and moon sponge. Then my ovaries, plus the tubes and my omentum that was also removed. Sadly everything had been sliced during the biopsy. However, I was able to put the pieces of my ovaries back together, once more smudging, praying and letting go. I was giving thanks for my miraculous body, thanks for the babies my ovaries had helped to produce, and honouring these creative organs that lived inside me for forty eight years. These organs that brought me so much wisdom, the wisdom of my female hormones, my wise blood, my wise body, my wise womb. I was also honouring my ancestors, and my matrilineal line, asking that these offerings be accepted and transformed by our Earth Mother, and by my ancestors.

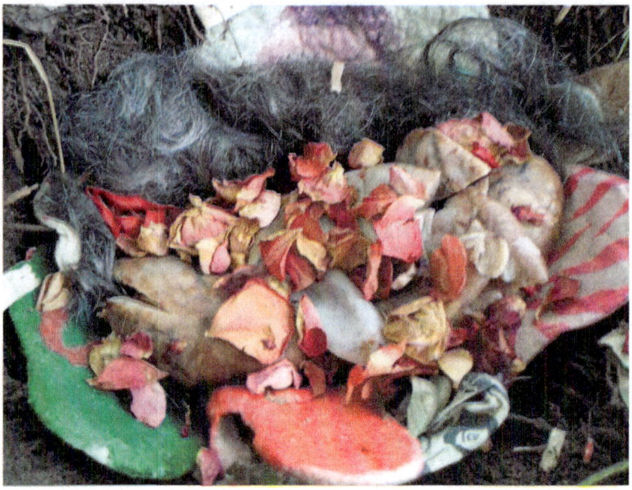

Letting go, letting go, letting go.... Sprinkling them with rose petals gathered by myself and friends over the summer....Rest in peace ovaries. You served me well.

This is how we reclaim surgery: make it sacred, make it ritual, make it yours.

This round of chemo knocks me for six. The steroids keep me going for a couple of days, even though the nausea kicks in pretty fast. By day three there's deep ache in the core of my bones, shooting pains, night sweats, day time hot flushes, night shivers, and insomnia. A strong desire to give up and die while my body is fighting for it's life. I have constant nausea, gut pain, burning pain, and a feeling of being slowly poisoned to death. During this week all the grief around my friend Sally's death also rose up.

As much as I'm attempting to see 'chemo as love', my mental health is being challenged to the core by the desperate feelings my body is going through.

This round I picked up the book by Eve Ensler (she is now called V) "In the Body of the World" (I even found a signed second hand copy!), in which she writes her vulnerable story of having uterine cancer and the gruelling surgery and chemo. This is woven around her memoirs of childhood, abuse, her work with war crime survivors, the Vagina Monologues, along with her relationship with her body, addiction and the creation of the City of Joy in the Congo. Wow, this is a powerful book and was a huge comfort to me while I was in the depths of despair.

Eve's therapist suggested she see the chemo as Kali energy, burning away all her trauma, including all the women's stories she's heard; all that needs to go, so she can be born anew. A Phoenix from the flames. Yes, I think I'll use that image for the next round! I have decided to request a lower dose this time, and possibly have a break after we see what the scan (due the following month) shows.

Prior to starting treatment I had a couple of phone appointments with the doctors at the Penny Brohn cancer centre. They were great, and really practical, while also used to dealing with patients who were combining natural healing, diet and lifestyle changes in to their healing protocol. They gave me loads of advice, and one thing that stuck in my mind was that 'I was in charge' and that I could ask for the drug doses to be lowered, changed etc. It was my body and I had a right to stop treatment or insist on changes. This really helped me feel empowered going into the choice to take chemo.

So I call my chemo doctor and explain how awful I've been feeling (laying it on thick- the dark thoughts and all) and that I want to try a lower dose. By this time he's got the scan results. It's good news, the tumour in my womb has shrunk by 50%, so he's encouraging me STRONGLY to continue with the current dose, since it's working. Mmmm, it's difficult to argue with that. I tell myself it's a short term fix for long term results and agree to stay on the high dose.

I know it's so hard for loved ones to witness me going though such pain. There's really nothing much to be done but offer kisses, hugs, hot water bottles, mint tea, suggestions of rubbish TV to distract me- and to keep offering food just incase it might be the day I feel like eating.

Tom has to take a week off work to support me through the days post chemo, and, life more or less gets cancelled for the family as I need constant care. By day five I managed to be driven to acupuncture which is proving to be another life -line. My acupuncturist has explained the five elements and how chemo is basically out to destroy everything, including me and my Spirit. When he looked into my eyes and said "Where's Rachael gone?" I almost cried.

When I described how I'd been feeling he was on it. He smoothed and cleared my liver energy, showing me points to strengthen my Spirit energy at home, basically working on bringing back my FIRE, because when my Spirit is strong, I can deal with anything!

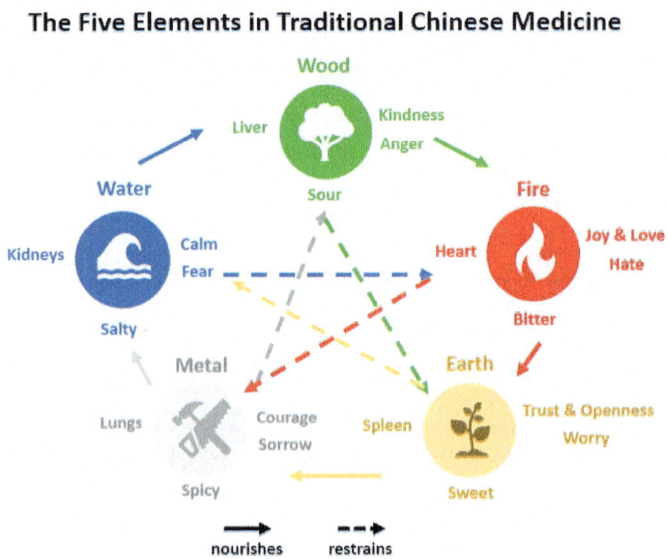

The five elements all feed one another. Chemo totally breaks this cycle- hence the body, mind, emotions and spirit all feel dreadful.

By day eight I felt strong enough to make a video, reading from the last chapter of The Body of the Earth. These writings feel very relevant in these times as we go though the world's changes. We need to stay resilient, stay strong in our circles, be prepared to lose everything, and despite it all RISE!

So this becomes my new monthly routine. Some months chemo is postponed, due to my bloods showing low white blood cells. I'm always relieved and see it as a week to focus deeper on healing. More time for walks in nature, listening to uplifting meditations. I've been listening to Abraham Hicks "mash up's"- His quotes set to music! Great to stick on my headphones while I stomp in the woods. More green juices. More REST! But for the rest of the family, their usual routine is thrown. Toms has taken a week off work which has to be rearranged. Luckily his boss is very understanding of our situation and is being as flexible as possible. We've arranged things for the children which need shifting around. It really is a lesson for all of us in going with the flow.

I have some ponderings on 'chemotherapy', noticing the word MOTHER in the middle

Che 'mother' apy

Let's break this word down. The 'chem' is the chemical aspect, and then there's the 'therapy', chemical therapy. So how about we reframe this? These days life feels like it's all about reframing! I'm gonna take the Che as Chi, Mother, therapy- energy medicine from the Mother. Beautiful!

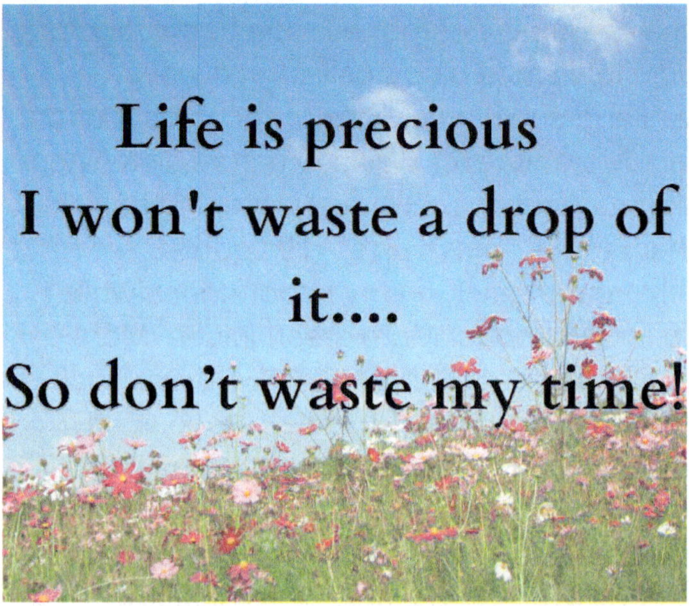

Outside in the world it's all 'Covid'. People are shocked when they hear I'm travelling to Stroud for the mistletoe. It's interesting to see how many people are interpreting these 'lock down rules', since I am allowed to travel for appointments, and I actually enjoy the fact the roads are quiet!

I observed all the, what I call 'nonsense' in the world, from a very different perspective. By choosing life I was choosing to live every day as an adventure. Every day I was waking up, living with a serious cancer diagnosis. I'd faced death, decided to live life, and no way was I going to let anyone tell me what I could and couldn't do!

We had decided to take the children out of school when they closed and moved education to on-line. They were at a Steiner School and our parenting philosophy was to not have them on screens, so to start using that wasn't in alignment for us.

It seemed crazy that at my friends funeral we were only 'allowed' a certain number of people (even though it was a beautiful outside service on a natural burial site) and people every where were cancelling 'life'. I was refusing to participate in any of it- I am free, I live free, and I'm alive (for now) so I will live my life, FULLY! This became part of my healing- what am *I choosing- to live or to die?*

I had chosen LIFE and was also choosing to live life in joy, as an adventure. Every day was an opportunity for fun, happiness and love!

So, despite the fear around me, along with the masks, the hand sanitising, the personal distancing- I did NONE of that- I hugged everyone happy to hug me as I knew that our bodies release oxytocin with every hug (that happy hormone!). I refused to wear a mask, as I would not have my oxygen supply restricted while I was healing, and I certainly wasn't going to add further toxic load to my body with chemical hand sanitisers. Interestingly- I didn't get ill- well apart from having stage 4 cancer! Haha. But then neither did any of my family or friends. Mmmm...ponder on that.

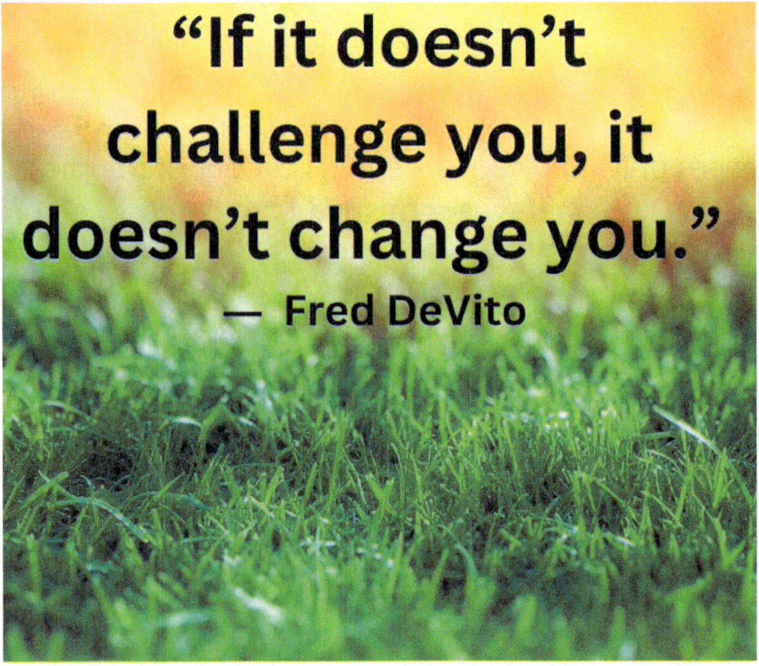

Fear and stress are massive factors in our health. So it's really something we need to look at and something I didn't look at enough first time round with cancer. Every day we are bombarded with stress and fear. I made a decision early on not to engage in any of the stuff the media was throwing at us, and also to protect my children, as it was another layer of stress I didn't need in my life while I was healing.

So let's fast forward. I finish the chemo, request a scan and I think I'll now have some rest and time to recover. But no, I start getting letters straight away about radiotherapy appointments- which I manage to hold off until the scan results come in.

Whenever I have a scan I try to let it go completely. I tell myself that there's no point worrying as I have no control over the outcome; the cancer has either grown or it hasn't. So let it go and deal with the results when they come in.

The day I get the phone call, it's January 2021. I've got a house full of home ed mums and children, so I'm 'shhhhhh-ing' them all while I talk. It's the nurse from radiology calling to book me in. I ask if my scan results have come in yet and she says "oh yes, no tumour in the womb or sign of cancer in the ligaments or anywhere else in the body". I ask her to repeat what she just said- "no tumour in the womb or sign of cancer in the ligaments or anywhere else in the body". So I reply, "well I'd like to just let that piece of news sink in, and no I wont be having radiotherapy thank you!"

I put the phone down and SCREAM- "I'm ALL CLEAR!!!!", the room is full of screaming, shouting, everyone jumping for joy, hugging me! Wow, I did it!

Afterwards, I did wonder how many people get signed up for radiotherapy without even checking what's going on with their cancer? If I hadn't asked about the scan, would they have told me I was all clear? I did later ask a nurse why, if I'm all clear would I need radiotherapy? Her reply was 'just in case'. So, I'm meant to put my body through that extreme treatment 'just in case' and without even giving it time to recover from the chemo? Well, I'm glad I said no. I'm glad I had a very clear gut feeling of "I'm done!" And I know in my bones that I am DONE and

I'm on the GOLDEN TIMELINE OF RADIANCE!

Chapter 3

Navigating Expectations from others. Seeking social, emotional, alternative and professional support. Dancing the divide.

When Family and Friends Can't Support Your Choices.

One of the hardest things when we choose not to go the allopathic route is the reaction of friends and family.

Of course, they love us and want the best for us, and most people have a negative experience of cancer- we all know people who have died from it.

My father died of leukaemia back in 2009. I always wondered if it was the leukaemia that he died of, or the chemo?

In fact it was my fathers diagnosis that got me looking into natural therapies and diet, including reading Kris Carr's books and watching the Truth about Cancer films. They gave me the foundations of my that belief cancer can be healed.

For the most part I was supported in my decision. But the odd few were pressuring me to have surgery, so I bought them the book Radical Remission. At the same time I maintained very strong boundaries. I would not be bullied or emotionally manipulated into surgery. I was also straight talking; "if you can't support me, then please don't contact me."

I feel most are coming from their own place of fear. It takes a lot to put your own fear aside and support someone, and it also takes a lot to acknowledge and hold compassion for those who are stuck in fear and can't see another way. But there is another way; many people are healing from cancer and living happy healthy lives with cancer! That's what Radical Remission is all about.

Dr. Kelly A. Turner, founder of the Radical Remission Project, has uncovered nine factors that can lead to a spontaneous remission from cancer—even after conventional medicine has failed.

From her research she found seventy five factors that could account for the healing, nine of these factors occurred with the greatest frequency, as outlined in her book;

Changing your diet.

Taking control of your health.

Following your intuition.

Using herbs and supplements.

Releasing suppressed emotions.

Increasing positive emotions.

Embracing social support.

Deepening your spiritual connection.

Having strong reasons for living.

I bought several copies of this book and passed it around friends and family, who were open to learning more.

When we face a threshold in life- whatever it is- an illness, a death, changing job, leaving home, at "mid life", starting school/college, having a baby.... SUPPORT is VITAL!

There's a saying "it takes a village to raise a child". I would say we all need a village- no matter what.

And calling in your village is one of the first pieces of advice I give folks who are newly diagnosed. In fact, it's advice I give everyone! Call in your village and let the love in. I find plenty resist this. They don't feel worthy, or that they deserve help. They don't want to be the centre of attention, they don't want to 'seem needy'...the excuses are endless! Part of calling in your support is allowing people to love you, and to love yourself.

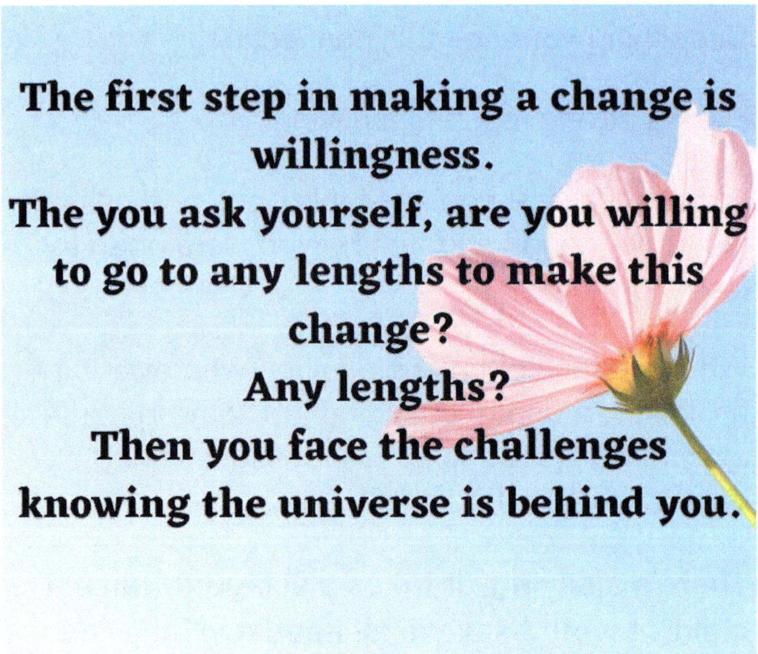

This cancer initiation is an initiation of LOVE! Many of those diagnosed aren't living a full life. Sometimes they don't have any love or enthusiasm for life, while many have experienced trauma, hardships, and massive difficulties and are just about getting through life.

Then cancer comes and forces you to stop, re-asses, look at what's not working and CHOOSE LIFE! The alternative is that you keep going, head down, refusing to look at anything or make changes… we can all guess where that takes you.

ASK YOURSELF THE QUESTIONS-

DO I WANT TO LIVE?

AND

WHAT DO I WANT TO LIVE FOR?

For some reason I've spent my life deep in work work surrounding 'self help'. I read Louise Hay when I was in my teens, spent my twenties reading all the old classics- Men are from Mars, Families and How to Survive Them, Creative Visualisation. I had shelves and shelves of these type of books! Addiction recovery work, and leading workshops from my twenties through to my forties. These are all tools that have stood me in good stead over the last couple of years.

I've deepened my self-love (and self- care), I've opened to allow others to love me more. I've chosen to really LOVE LIFE. Even on days when life isn't so great, I look for the opportunities for LOVE and service! Every day I'm grateful for the day, for another day to grow. Each day is a rebirth, a day to choose LIFE.....

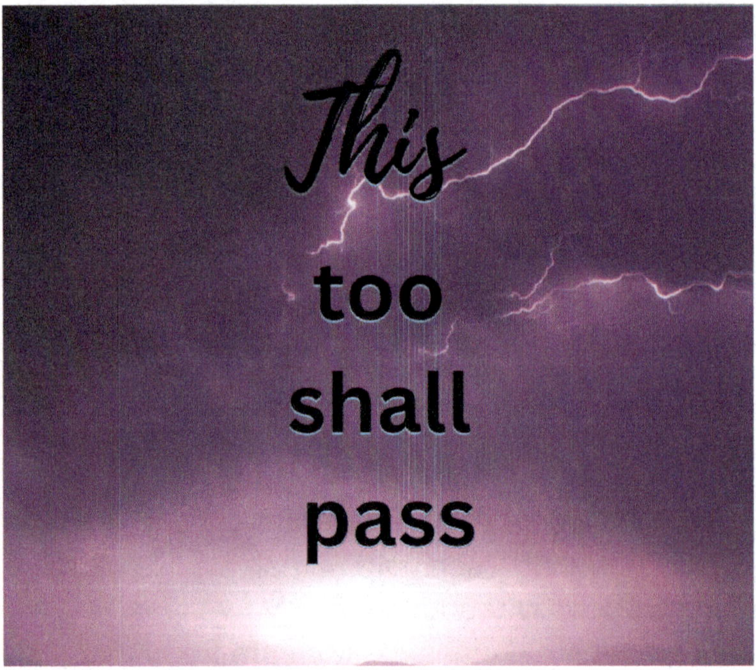

Each morning in my meditation I focus on LOVE - everything just IS love! Even the chemotherapy drugs are LOVE if you choose to see them that way.

In every moment you can change your mind about anything and make it work for you!

Meditate and Breathe, Surrender to what is. Face Death.

After my diagnosis I did more meditation and breath work than ever before. There are many reasons to choose these practices. Of course the number one is that they support you in de-stressing. The body relaxes, and doing breath work brings more oxygen into the body, which is the enemy of cancer. It helps you feel more energised and, more balanced and the 'side effect' I hadn't considered was that it helped me have more *acceptance* of my illness and the possibility of death.

Ultimately, no one has the answers or any guarantees, either- about healing cancer or anything else. Yes, doctors have statistics to back up their treatments, and we hear stories of people who get well from certain protocols. But who knows what will work for us? Even though I had faith in a miracle and trusted the protocols I was using, there was always a little doubt that it wouldn't work, that I might die. When that doubt crept in, I would go and meditate and breathe. I would surrender, let go and find that place inside myself where I felt love, safety and vibrancy.

From this place, I knew even if I died, all was well.

By facing death, surrendering to it, I discovered I wasn't scared to die. In fact, I came to believe that there is no death, just a change of state- which is where meditation and breath work can take you!

Yes, there is grief, grief to leave behind my family, friends, and loved ones. But I also felt lucky to be able to process this while I could. Anyone who dies suddenly or while crippled with pain doesn't have a chance to look at life, to review, grieve, and prepare. I was able to discuss with my family where I would like to be buried, to write my will and think about all my friends and the gifts I would leave them. It wasn't an easy process, but I managed it with the tools of meditation, breath, tuning into my deep inner wisdom.

With facing death there comes a freedom; I don't think anyone is truly free until they face their own mortality. Something in me has changed. I don't take life for granted any more, or so seriously. I let go of all the 'stuff' that I felt was holding me back. I trust more in life, in the flow of life and, in the synchronicities that the Universe shows me.

Right at the start of my diagnosis, I began to notice synchronicities- signs that I took to mean that I was on the right path, that everything was going to be okay. These gave me reassurance and comfort. While it's highly probable that those synchronicities had always been there, it took me slowing down, and letting go of the busyness of life, to start noticing them. These signs came in many forms, from literal words on the side of a van, to numbers repeating (I was seeing 333 a lot!!) to books that were passed on to me that contained just what I needed hear within the pages. I also found signs in nature such as, birds, heart-stones, and crystals.

For more on meditation and cancer I recommend You Can Conquer Cancer by Ian Gawlers

Chapter 4

Healing the wounded feminine-collective and individual. Trauma-collective and individual. Musings on Fear, Surrender. Life as a mirror.

It's interesting, isn't it how many women get cancer in our reproductive systems and our breasts; these deeply feminine parts of our bodies, that birth and nourish our children. On so many levels it's no surprise that these body parts are telling us about the imbalance of the masculine/feminine in the world.

Our breasts are like our Earth Mother, they nourish us as she does. But we have abused her, and abused women, abused our femininity and, our sexuality by posting breasts in newspapers, using them to sell cars, perfume, anything to make something 'sexy'. Our wombs are now cut open more often than not, births becoming more and more medicalised, but our wombs are longing for natural birth. Our cervix wants to dilate and open miraculously wide enough to birth a baby (talk to them both, I think you'll be surprised how chatty they are!), and then theres smear tests that personally I find traumatic and invasive (no matter how 'life saving' they are, it didn't save my life!) and then if your smear ain't 'normal'- let's just cauterise your cervix- no harm done with that eh? (see my interview with Kate Orsons about her post lletz trauma).

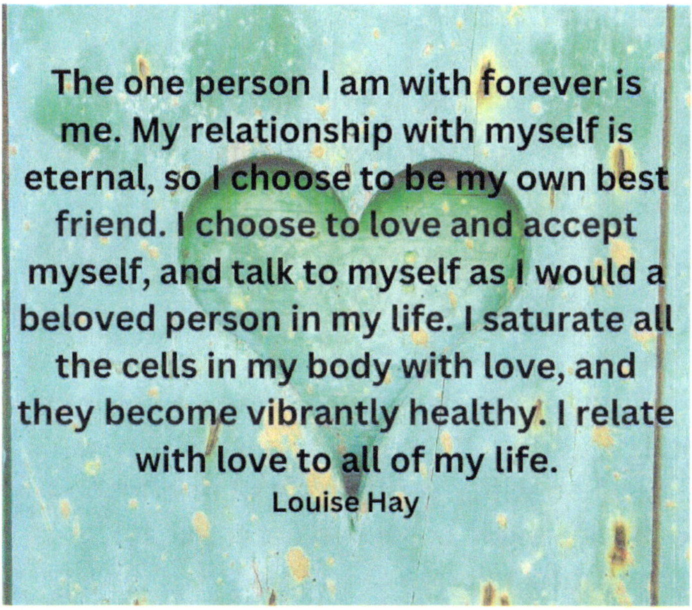

Our bodies are a mirror of what's going on in the world, so much so that when I was going through the chemo, having my cells annihilated, on my door-step the woods I walk were being felled, each stump brutally cut, churned up, the ground devastated. I would sit on those stumps marvelling at what was going on. What was happening here was being mirrored in my body, and yet what I witnessed was nature coming in to its glory. The following spring there would be more wild flowers than I had ever seen in these woods, while saplings would be popping up everywhere, along with the wild garlic. Then when it came to autumn, there would be so many fungi and mushrooms. This gave me such hope for my own recovery, that I could come back more wild than before!

Of course, when I was first diagnosed I was looking only to myself; what had I done to cause this, where in my her-story had it started? Was it sexual trauma, birth trauma, emotional trauma? Diet, poor nutrition, drinking tap water, bathing in tap water, lack of exercise? How much I smoked when I was younger, drank, and experimented with drugs? Was it because I was an empath? Had I picked up all the trauma of the women I had worked with over the years? And then eventually; is this collective trauma that I've taken into my body to heal?

We can never truly know the exact cause of cancer, most likely a combination of all of the above...

By the time I got to the 'secondary' diagnosis, I had stopped looking for causes. Really, why bother, you can't heal from the past. We heal by being totally in the present and knowing deep inside we're on the Golden Timeline Of Radiance NOW. I trusted my body to show me what I needed to do, and I trusted life to show me what I needed to do. Synchronicities, the 'right' person popping into my life, little nudges, healing dreams- they all presented themselves at the perfect time and I embraced the flow.

You can't heal from the past. We heal by being totally in the present and knowing deep inside we're on the Golden Timeline Of Radiance NOW.

I had quite an unusual response when the doctors told me I had cancer. I absolutely had no fear (shock yes- but no fear!). I knew I had the tools, support and inner guidance to get through this. And yes there were times that I did think 'getting through' might be dying.

The whole journey for me was a HUGE lesson in what surrender really is.

It's not just letting go – surrender is total trust, trust that if you jump, you'll be caught!

When the stage 4 diagnosis arrived and all the 'it's too late for treatment' from the doctors came at me, I had to dig really deep, to keep my faith, to feel the holding of the spirit world, to keep the knowing that everything would be okay, even when it wasn't!

I had to look Death deep in the eyes and say “if it's my time, then take me”, while also holding onto “I know it's not my time and I want to stay, I choose to stay”.

All through my healing I was holding these imbalances. Telling myself I was radiant and vibrant while feeling the tumours growing. I was affirming to myself 'I am perfect, God made me perfect, even with cancer, I am perfect.' Of course there were days doubts crept in. Days I cried and cried with grief that I may be leaving my children, that I may not see them growing up, having their own children, leaving my family and friends. Then I would surrender all over again knowing that God has a divine plan and trusting all will be well- whatever happens.

These ‘dark nights of the soul’ happened many times through the years of healing, sometimes coming out of nowhere. A song would trigger grief, or a conversation would bring up the 'cancer victim' story. But often they were linked with getting news from the doctor, or scan results, or even just before a scan. People call this scanxiety. It's totally normal. One part of me was being positive and convincing myself all was going to be okay, then the other was in total fear that the cancer may have spread and my mind was already speeding ahead to me being on my death-bed! Then in comes the surrender again.

Trust, what will be, will be, and whatever the outcome, I will be alright. In these times meditation was my best friend. Breathing calmed me, while meditation helped me surrender to what is, bringing joy into my heart and then taking action to move into joy- maybe dancing around the kitchen, or a walk in nature, seeing a friend...

More actions that needed to be taken concerned the practical things. Having been one of those who helps sort through a loved ones things after their death, I wanted to leave my own as clearly as possible. I started decluttering, and giving things away. I sold my business, wrote my will, and listed all my possessions and what would go to who. From this arose the need to do more forgiveness and letting go of more resentments that I didn't even know were still there, peeling back the layers until I was raw.

I visited a natural burial ground and cried and cried, deeply considering my final resting place for this body I am in was a much bigger process than I imagined it would be. People had said to me “well you're dead, so it doesn't matter where your body is, that's about those left behind and having a place they can visit”. But it was deeper than that for me, I wanted to honour this vessel I have walked through this life in and place her somewhere special. I just couldn't imagine being buried on land to which I had no connection and begged my husband to ask the local land owner about me being buried near my home. As it turned out, a very close friend passed and was buried on this natural site. So I accepted that I would be okay to be buried next to a dear sistar.

Sally's death came so suddenly. She had been my 'cancer sistar', even though her journey with breast cancer began before we met. She was given a secondary diagnosis not long after we connected and I was in awe of how she handled it, seeing cancer as a journey to love, self love, and love of life! In the years after I was diagnosed she rapidly deteriorated, cancer having spread to her spine and lungs and later her brain.

She had chosen not to do allopathic treatment until the last few years when she tried surgery, medications and injections, later chemo and radiotherapy. She passed away when I in the chemotherapy treatment, and I was so angry, and probably for the first time feeling scared- scared that these barbaric treatments I had agreed to wouldn't work.

I remember my son's little face (he was eight years old) when he heard that Sally had died, as he asked me if my treatments were going to work and all I could do was tell him "I hope so".

Then came another grappling with a 'dark night of the soul'. I had to do some serious self-talk assuring myself that this was MY Life, and my journey wasn't Sallys. We had different soul paths, we had lived different lives.... and eventually surrender once more to whatever was to be, was meant to be, even if that meant dying.

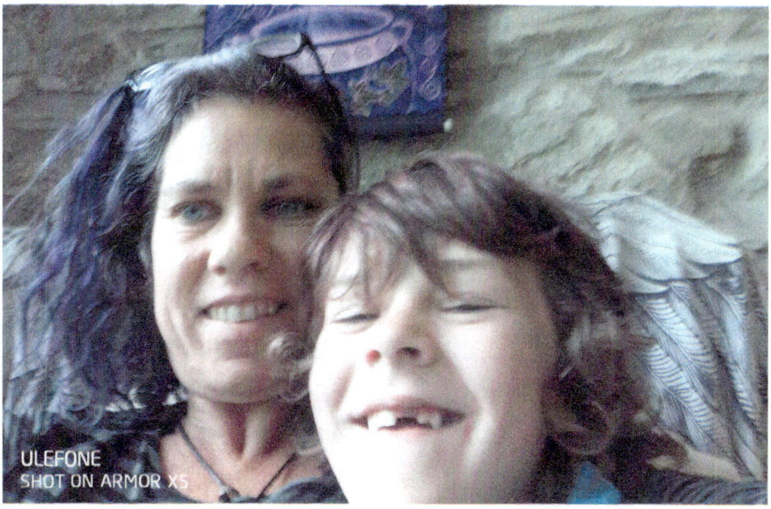

The anger- what was that about? I was angry Sally hadn't done more. She could have tried so many other protocols, that she had left it too late for treatment to work....yadda, yadda, yadda. Ultimately I had to accept she was gone, go into the grief of losing a friend and another layer of acceptance that everyone has free will to choose how to live and how to die.

I also want to mention here that death isn't failing- we all have to die some day! None of us know when our time is, or someone else's. If anything it's just a reminder to live well. Live the best life. Stay in joy! Sally totally taught me that. I've even heard famous yogis who have been diagnosed with cancer or terminal illness saying it is no failure to die and sometimes *something* has to kill us! We have this expectation that famous healers, yogis, masters live forever, that they will just breathe themselves slowly into death, but we all have our journey and we all have a soul contract, and for some of us it's just our time and that's just how it is. Life and death.

So while contemplating death, and facing death, surrendering to death, I was also passionately choosing Life! Making sure each day was an adventure, that days included joy, fun, beauty, and love. Whether that was hanging out with loved ones and friends, walks in nature and connecting to the earth and the trees, dancing to my favourite tunes, trips to Stroud for mistletoe therapy that included seeing old friends, or going to parties, sacred kirtans (chanting), and cacao ceremonies, drum circles....doing things that helped me feel *Alive*!

Having worked with many cancer thrivers over the last few years, I know my response to getting the cancer diagnosis was rare. Most people do have fear and I want to reassure you, it's okay to have fear…it's NORMAL to have fear…so don't try to deny it, run away from it….Fear is an absolutely natural and necessary feeling. It's part of our self-preservation and survival instinct that helps us to stay away from danger. We all have our fears, things such as spiders, the dark, snakes, and death. Most are ungrounded and projected by our mind and emotions, such as the fear of loneliness, and losing a job or a spouse…. These can take over to a place where fear is controlling our behaviours, choices and therefore our lives. This kind of fear has a strong negative knock-on effect on our physical and mental health.

So, let's look at how we can resolve, make peace and move beyond fear…

When you can identify fear, you are half way there to making peace with it…and TRUST, this too will pass….

Know that eventually your diagnosis will be come a 'normal' part of your life and the fear will just disappear.

Things that help support moving out of fear.

Listen to positive stories of people who have healed and those who live happy healthy lives with cancer. Examples include Kris Carr, Louise Hay, Wayne Dyer, and Anita Moorjani.

Reprogram those fearful thoughts. For example, if a fearful thought comes in (such as “no, I can’t do that”) identify it, and then replace with a new thought, such as “Of course I can do it, I will figure it out, I will be okay.”

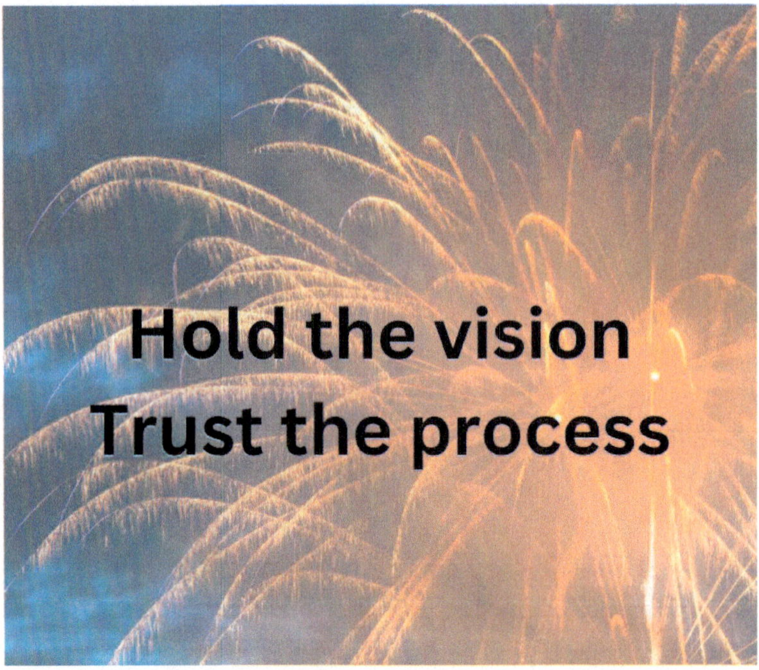

Use all the tools available to you to support healing. I love EFT (there are loads of videos on YouTube), and TRE (Trauma Release Exercises) helps move stuck emotions out of your body. I would recommend learning this under a practitioner, of whom there are many across the world. Find a form of exercise that works for you, (yoga, tai chi, running, a walk in nature). We are all different and different things help promote calm!

Find a faith; believe in something bigger than you. Twelve Step programmes have successfully supported addicts out of chronic addiction by suggesting they find a 'Higher Power', which then becomes their defence against picking up the next drug/drink. The same concept can be used for ANYTHING!

If you really want to release fear from your life, find a belief in something outside of yourself. Just choose something.... God, the universe, love, your higher self, your ancestors, guides....it really doesn't matter what word you use; when you believe in something bigger than yourself, it allows you to feel supported, loved and protected.

When we start to believe in something bigger than ourselves it is easier to switch our small, limited, fear based thinking into something more open, loving and supportive.

When we shift out of fear based thinking- into abundant, loving thinking, our life shifts to a new level and it will feel easier and more natural to live from our highest purpose.

Faith replaces fear.

I love the movie- The Shift- by Wayne Dyer. See if you can find it online.

Chapter 5

Ritual and Ceremony and spiritual warriorship. Connecting with Nature, Cosmos, Heart and Soul. Are we on our own? Working with the invisible world of spirit, ancestors prayer/journeying/healing/meditation/visualisation/circles/quantum/affirmations/intentions

All through my story, and this book, I have shared some of the ceremonies and rituals that supported me along the way. Whilst you can create your own special ceremonies and rituals, my aim is to live life as a sacred ceremony, in gratitude and presence.

These are some of the ceremonies I used during my Cancer journey. I honoured my moontime blood and my river baptism with my community of women. They gathered to make me a blanket, circling with them while they spoke about me and the impact I'd had on their lives (that was emotional), as well as the gifts they made me as support talismans while I was in hospital. Having my body painted and sung to in our Red Tent, friends and family holding me during my surgery with drumming, prayers, song....burying my ovaries in a post-surgery ritual.

If I hadn't had the faith that I'd developed over years of working the twelve step programme I might have struggled to feel completely held by spirit. But who knows, maybe I would have found my way? I also know that through my addiction recovery, I had seen miracles, including 'hopeless' cases turn their lives around. So I knew a miracle was possible. I was one of those miracles- from chronic addict to staying clean and sober for over twenty years!

Surrendering to healing was all I could do. I didn't want to 'fight' cancer, as it felt like fighting myself. After all the cancer was part of me, so how could I heal if I was fighting myself? And this word ‘fighting’ is also like ‘willpower’ for me. Many people say ‘oh I don’t have the willpower’ and as far as I’m concerned my willpower took me to the wrong places! My willpower was definitely going against the flow, going against life, fighting.

Ultimately it was surrendering, surrendering to life, surrendering to death, surrendering to my higher power, my higher self, Source, which enabled me to find peace and in the peace we become whole. **I became whole.**

Why do we choose that language when dealing with illness? Things like 'battling cancer, fighting cancer?' Words are spells; we have to be aware how we use them. When people would ask "I hear you're battling cancer?" I would reply- "No, I'm loving the cancer, loving it well". I was also conscious not to say "my cancer, or my illness" I didn't want to own it; I didn't want it to become my story. How many people do you know who become 'Cancer Mary', 'Cancer Ben', "Oh you know, Abby -who has Breast Cancer", or "John, you know John- with the prostate cancer?" When we start to be labelled or label ourselves we take on the story.

So many friends said to me I should go into working with women with cervical cancer, I could be the 'Cervix Whisperer/Shaman/Healer'. But I didn't want to. I knew I had more to offer. I knew that healing was about wholeness, not just focussing on one bit of us! After thirty years of focussing on the womb, I'd learned that lesson!

Intuition is key. Your intuition will guide you.

To step fully into healing ourselves, we need to become our own Spiritual Warrior, which will be whatever the word 'spiritual' means for you. I know many people who just used reiki to heal, or prayer, fasting, and breath work. You just have faith in whatever is your 'thing'. However you have to know '*your thing*'. We can't heal by copying what someone else has done, because we all have our own path. Intuition is key. Your intuition will guide you.

My intuition guided me into churches where I knelt and wept- praying for healing. It lead me to work with shamanic healing, to books with healing meditations and visualisations. It led me to psychics and channellers. Most importantly, all of these paths resonated deeply in my soul, and led me deeper into myself, into my own heart, into my own life of Joy, Beauty and Love.

Connecting with nature was a huge part of my healing. I had been connecting with the Earth as my Mother for such a long time. Whilst my mum and I have a good relationship now, there were years where it was difficult, particularly in my teens and twenties, when I became a teen mum and left home. At that time I had to learn to mother myself while mothering my children. Without the nurturing mother that I believed I had needed as a child, I adopted Mother Earth as my Mama and my role model. I now know that my mum was the perfect mother for me in this incarnation, and that my soul choose her very carefully for the job! But back then it was a very different story- I had been a 'sensitive' child and was needy and clingy. Unfortunately as the third child in the family there wasn't a lot of time for my neediness, hence I had to learn that 'no one was coming to save me' and I had to self soothe. I guess this is part of my story of being drawn into drugs and addiction so young. I found the world an overwhelming place to be- until I learned that my sensitivities were my super power and didn't need to be numbed; I could gradually feel the feelings and be okay!

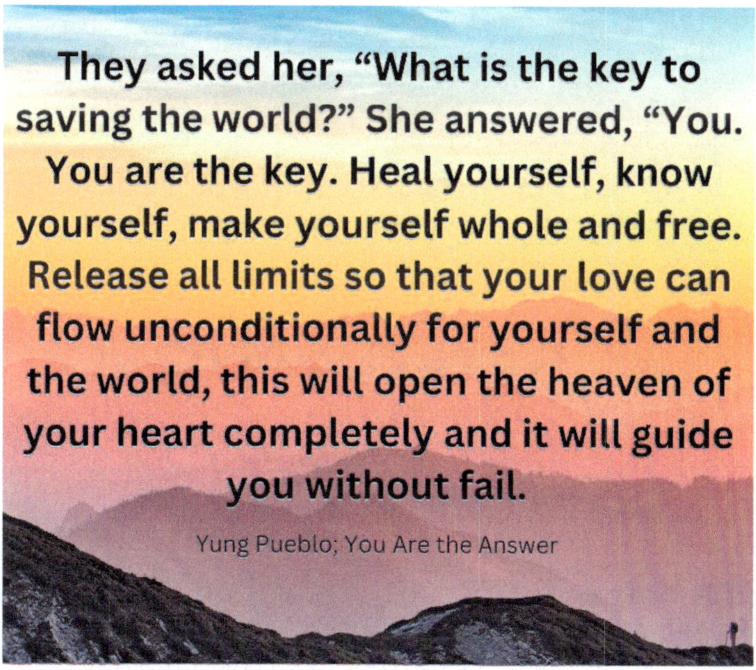

I totally believe the Earth and nature hold healing energies, so most days I would get outside, put my yoni directly on to the earth, and breathe her in through my cervix. I also visited the Callanish Stones on the isle of Lewes in Scotland. These seem to have a 'womb' stone, with even cervix.

So each visit to the stones I sat on the 'cervix stone' and prayed for healing. Trees are a love of mine too. I'm sure the oxygen they release has healing properties so I would walk in the woods, taking deep breaths, imagining the air coming into my body was sparkly, magical, and healing. I would also do forest bathing before I even knew what that was.

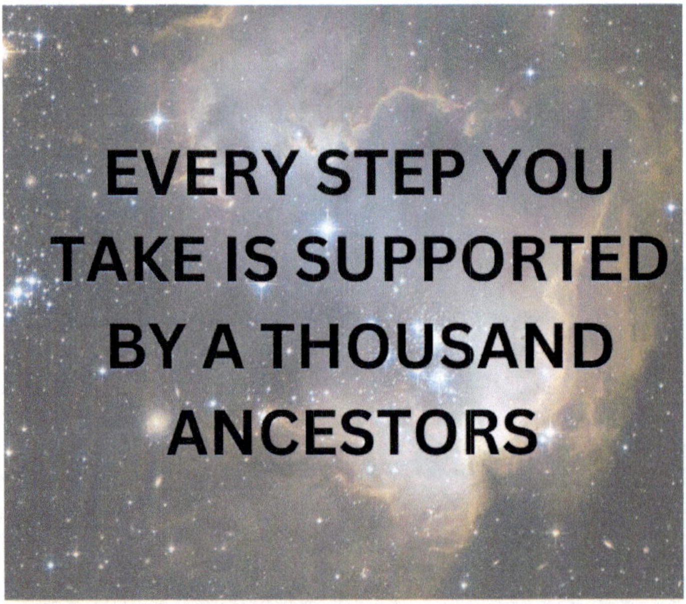

Do you remember from my diagnosis chapter I had mentioned there being a peace and calmness in the room when I was told I had cancer? It was an interesting experience as my friend who was with me also felt a calming energy and wondered at the time if there was an angelic presence in the room.

The mystery unfolded several months later when I had a Quantum EFT session (I go more into EFT in my Healing Manifesto chapter later in the book. Do check it out EFT it's a wonderful healing tool!) In this session, not only were we tapping through what was going on for me in that present time, the practitioner suggested using the 'quantum' to go back in time to the moment of diagnosis, as she imagined that this must have been a shocking and traumatic moment and to tap through that. I did explain to her that actually I had felt very calm and even said about feeling an angelic presence in the room with me.

Anyway, we proceeded to re-imagine this scenario except this time imagining I'm in the room with myself. I am tapping the EFT points on the me who is receiving the diagnosis - am I the angelic presence in the room???

Whilst this felt very beautiful, it also blew my mind that I could 'time travel' and support myself. Well this opens up a whole new level of healing, and reminded something at my core about using distance healing across space and time. This isn't really a new experience for me as I remembered as a child having what I thought were angelic visitations, only to realise when I got into inner child healing many years ago that those angelic visits were actually my future self coming to reassure little me that everything was going to be okay. I think the only way my child brain could make sense of these visits was to create the future me as an angel.

Of course at the time of doing this work, I had no idea I was doing quantum healing. I have another similar story which only dawned on me when I was coming out of a deep walking meditation on the week with Dr Joe. I was thinking back to my sorry state in my addiction days and thinking how grateful I was to be clean and sober and living an amazing life now. I felt called to speak to that lost part of me and tell her to stop the self-abuse, and to tell her I loved her and that in order for her to become me, she needed to change- and make big changes. I kept reassuring her that I loved her and that everything was going to be fine, and that she would become me, standing here, in the sun, feeling amazing!

What had actually happened back on that dark night in 2002 was that I was lying on the ground in a mess after falling off my bike (drunk cycling!) and I had a vision of an angel reaching out her hand. She was telling me she loved me but that it was time to change. I had important work to do here and I needed to clean up. Every time I think of that, I well up. All those times it was me being my own guardian angel. For years in recovery rooms I told the story of the angel pulling me out of the gutter -literally!

As for other 'spirits', I have some pretty special stories about encounters with Mary Magdalene. The first took place on my way home after an acupuncture session (not long after my first diagnosis) and I had an inner nudge to take a left turn and head to a nearby Chapel. All I new about it was that it contained ancient ogham carvings and had a very old stone Celtic cross in the grave yard. I went inside and wandered around, looking at the ogham carvings and reading the little pamphlet about the church. I lit a prayer candle and knelt at the altar and said a prayer for myself. That was when the flood gates opened, I cried, and cried, and cried. I did all the “why me, why now, I don't want to die....what about my children, I want to live for my children”. All the emotions I'd been bottling inside me came tumbling out. Eventually, they subsided and I wandered outside feeling calm. I walked around the graves and spotted the Celtic cross, and was about to leave when I noticed a yew tree with a sign by it saying ‘The Bleeding Yew’. I could see that it had red sap dripping on one side of its trunk. I put some onto my forehead and sat with my back to the trunk, closed my eyes and felt into it’s energy. In my mind’s eye, I saw Mary Magdalene standing in front of me. She smiled and told me that the yew would be my medicine, and that I should take some of her needles home and make medicine. I’m well aware that Yew is a powerful tree, and that it's poisonous, but- what I didn't know is that it is also the source the cancer drug Tamoxifen! I made a gentle tree essence from the few small fallen branches I took home which felt like the right way to use this 'medicine' gift from the Yew.

After this I felt Mary (and Yeshua and Mother Mary) with me pretty much every day, supporting my healing. I would see Mary bending over my womb with her hands on me, sending healing light into me, sometimes blowing her sacred breath in to me. Yeshua and Mother Mary were always by her side. The next time Mary stepped in strongly was while I was having a sound healing;- the sound practitioner also felt her presence. Mary urged me to look more deeply at my father line and open up to the healing of my father. This was way before my realisation about the story I was carrying about my dads death and his chemotherapy treatment, so I struggled a little to piece this together. But after this healing I felt my father around me much more strongly than before, always encouraging and reassuring me and saying it wasn't my time to die.

All through having cancer and treatment I called on my angels and guides daily. The evening healing prayer to the angels I used was from a Caroline Myss book, which is in the next section. I used visualisations where angels took me to healing temples. My guides worked on my body and held me though tough emotions, while my spirit animals accompanied me and gave me comfort. When I had doctors appointments and scans, I called on my angels and guides to calm me. Whilst I imagine this could all sound very strange to someone who isn't on familiar terms with angels, guides and spirit animals, I can assure you they are all very real to me. I feel them step into my energy field and instantly my energy shifts.

I also worked with my ancestor line. I felt it was important to call in my ancestors as this was a huge clearing for them too. All the work I was doing was repairing, mending, healing old and future family patterns. I remember being told in my twenties by a clairvoyant that I would be the one in my family to break unhealthy family patterns- I always wondered why I was chosen, why not my older siblings? Well the answer is clear- I'm the only one of my siblings to have children. So of course, I have to break the generational patterning for my children and future grandchildren.

I had a session after all my treatment had finished with a psychic who told me all my ancestors where gathered around and had all hung lanterns in a tree, symbolising the love and light they were holding for me; hundreds of lanterns were in this tree, just for me. It was an overwhelming thought, but also a huge comfort to know my ancestors where with me and 'had my back'.

Daily morning meditations became part of my routine. I had got into the habit of working with Dr Joe Dispenza's meditations (I had read some of his books so knew about his own miraculous healing). I found many people I met on the more 'natural' healing cancer forums were mentioning his Blessing the Energy Centres meditations/ visualisations, so I had downloaded a few, as well as some of his others. I really love the walking meditations- particularly 'Walking into your Future'.

I was finally getting that healing is about change. Nothing changes unless we change; change your story, change you life. **Healing is a FEELING**- it's about feeling whole, feeling joy, and feeling a love for life!

And as I mentioned, I found there was a Dr Joe week in London coming up- I knew tickets sold like hot cakes so I just surrendered and trusted the money would come and if I was meant to be there, I would get one of those 'golden tickets'! And I did, and the money came. I had a huge donation from my wonderful friend Gill, whose partner was also at this time on a cancer journey (sadly as I write this in November 2022 he has passed away). I was also given many smaller ones that added up to the cost of the ticket. Now I needed to get strong so I could attend as it was scheduled for November 2020. Then, with all the Covid stuff it was postponed. Although this was a disappointment, the reality was that in November 2020 I was on my third round of chemo and would have struggled to be there. So I trusted the divine timing. It was rescheduled, cancelled again and rescheduled, until finally it took place in August 2022 when I was well, vital and totally ready to shake up my life! All I can say is that, if you get the opportunity to go to a week or a weekend with Dr Joe, then do it. It's a life changing experience. It was epic and like being in biblical times- people being healed all over the room!

I would say Dr Joe is a modern day mystic, he balances science with spiritual, he proves the spiritual with science!

I made video diaries each day which you can watch on my blog. I had many insights and 'mystical' experiences while I was there, seeing HUGE beings – Masters and Angels supporting the healing sessions we did on the last three days. I had a conversation with my dad that was a massive revelation. I time travelled to my past self and experienced another meeting with Mary Magdalene, Yeshua, Mother Mary, Isis, and was downloaded with my 'full soul'. That story is in my Mary Magdalene on line course.

The after effects of taking part in this week are still rippling through my life. Each morning I'm reminding myself of the feeling of being in such a large group (2.5k!) meditating together, and feeling my wholeness, my peace, and seeing my future self- happy and free. Visualising the whole world in a state of love and light, peace and unity- happy and free.

My video diaries from the Dr Joe week can be found on my Hello Cervix blog.

Affirmations and intentions are also a part of my healing, although I did struggle to affirm my health when I could feel cancer growing inside me. So I changed to using words like vital, vitality, radiant, radiance, whole, wholeness, peace, growth, and change. I took my focus off my healing and onto my feelings, my energy, my state of being; if I could be whole, and feel whole, then everything was fine. It really is about changing your energy. How do we do that? Read on...

I used words like vital, vitality, radiant, radiance, whole, wholeness, peace, growth, and change.

As part of my healing I read Sophie Sabbage's book The Cancer Whisperer. I felt blessed to have a few group zoom sessions with her. She was as feisty as me and really got you to look at where you really didn't want to look! After working with her she said to the group "Rachael is a Spiritual Warrior- coming at her healing from the spiritual holding of the twelve steps." Reading Sophie's books I could feel her own knowledge of the twelve step spiritual programme entwined into her own work.

"Rachael is a Spiritual Warrior" Sophie Sabbage

Change your energy!

From the cancer people I have worked with, it seems there are two types of cancer patients:

The first one is willing to do everything to beat cancer and believes their purpose on earth isn't over yet.

The other unfortunately withdraws from society and waits for the inevitable end.

If you or someone you know has been diagnosed with cancer. It's perfectly normal to be shocked, surprised, or scared. If you can allow the fear and shock to run though your body, releasing it and remembering that this is your body's way of *'waking you up to changing your life*!'

To all those who say- cancer won't change their lives- cancer SHOULD change your life. This is why it appears! Whatever you were doing before wasn't working for you- otherwise cancer wouldn't have come. It's time to make BIG CHANGES!

At the very beginning, I made a decision to live with cancer. This choice is totally going against the mainstream tide, which is at times uncomfortable and lonely. That's why its super important you have your supportive tribe around you. I knew that cancer could be nuked, poisoned and cut out, but I also knew that these days many people live with stable cancer in their bodies. i.e. The cancer isn't taking over. So I decided that I would befriend cancer, give it a home, and love myself into health.

I chose not to fear cancer, but to love it, to heal from the inside.

All dis-ease is just your body needing something, some sort of attention and change.

Cancer is the biggest call to get your attention and the biggest call to change!

I made changes, day by day. This way the little changes become big ones. Take small steps, because the bigger picture of what needs to change is overwhelming.

So, just change one thing at a time; baby steps.

Do what's manageable. I was healing myself while being a mum, running a business, going through menopause; if I can do it, so can you!

Cancer means having to put yourself first- your well-being is the most important thing here. So sorry kids, sorry friends, sorry family!

This is all about YOU.

It's time to stop doing the stuff you don't want to do, and definitely no more people pleasing!

Life is precious, don't waste a drop!

So what does it mean to change your energy? When I woke up every day I would pop on my headphones and go straight into a Dr Joe Dispenza Meditation (I recommend his Blessing the Energy Centres ones and his book Becoming Supernatural.) So I was beginning my morning with my heart open, and excited for the adventure of the day.

I would also pray. I'm not a Christian but I do believe in the power of prayer and that our guides, ancestors and angels are waiting to help us- we just need to ask! So I suggest finding a prayer that feels right for you. It could be as simple as 'please help', or use a traditional prayer. I like one of the prayers from the Twelve Step programme. This is the Step three prayer-

God, (or use the word Light, Love, Mother, Source, Universe....)

I offer myself to Thee

To build with me and to do with me as Thou wilt.

Relieve me of the bondage of self, that I may better do Thy will.

Take away my difficulties,

That victory over them may bear witness

To those I would help of Thy Power,

Thy love and Thy way of life,

May I do Thy will always!

I fell in love with Tosha Silvers writings and philosophy. Her books include Outrageous Openness: Letting the Divine Take the Lead and

Change Me Prayers: The Hidden Power of Spiritual Surrender.

A Change Me Prayer is fundamentally a prayer from your ego to your Divine Self. Tosha says it's the answer to the question "How do you change a pattern that is persistent and that you've tried everything you know of to change?"

A Change Me Prayer goes like this:

Divine Beloved, please change me into someone who is willing to receive.

Divine Beloved, please change me into someone who can deeply and sincerely surrender my will to THY will and truly TRUST the Divine to take the lead.

Divine Beloved, please change me into someone who truly knows her value and worth. I am yours, you are mine, we are One.

Tosha's teaching about 'letting the Divine take the lead' is life changing. But in our crazy culture (which brainwashes us into thinking we should be able to manifest whatever we want by making the right list, taking the right actions, and doing the right affirmations), it can be very difficult for the ego to let go of the reins.

Change Me Prayers are sooooo helpful and practical for learning to trust ourselves and remove ourselves from the traps of our ego. I believe the Divine has a plan for each of us, our destiny, our sacred blueprint (or gold print as I like to call it). We chose this before we were born. Our Divine Higher Self is inside us and talking to us constantly. Our job is to align with that plan and let it lead us. Few of us have been taught to listen for this guidance! The basic Change Me Prayer is: "Please change me into someone who trusts the Divine part of myself."

This takes practice, and over time you'll find that it works.

Letting our Higher Self/Divine take the lead doesn't mean you sit around and wait for God to do it all. It means you remain open to the messages, synchronicities and inner prompting you receive and then take action on what you're shown.

You could simply say "Make use of me today". Then whatever comes your way, you look at it as an opportunity to be of service. This also takes your focus off yourself, because with cancer its very easy to become obsessed with your own health and wellbeing!

This may seem contradictory to what I was saying earlier about putting yourself first earlier- and it's important to maintain balance and keep your cup full- it's that saying- you can't give from an empty cup! But there is a difference between doing the work of the Divine, and just spreading yourself too thin. While on my healing path, my 'divine work' showed up as conversations in shops. I would over hear someone talking about a diagnosis, or a friend with cancer, and I would get a 'divine nudge' to tell them what I was doing. Or it was taking another cancer buddy for a session at the oxygen centre, or for an infra-red sauna, and just listening to them and how their healing journey was going. It was educating the different practitioners and doctors I was under that it was a matter of going with the flow and trusting the Divine would use me!

I also prayed at night, every night before putting my head on the pillow, and asked for my body to be healed in my sleep.

I used this prayer from Carolyn Myss' book- Intimate Conversations with the Divine:

"LORD, SEND YOUR HEALING angels to me tonight. Escort me out of my body and into the healing realm. Grant that they may repair my depleted soul, my weary body, and my burdened heart. May they clear the illusions from my mind and awaken me to what I need to see clearly about myself—my own actions, and all that I need to repair within myself. Let me rest in the silence of the celestial realm, calm in the company of angels as they heal what I am unable to heal due to my own limitations. Let their healing graces remain in my system and illuminate my thoughts with insight, my heart with love, and my body with stamina—that I might continue to serve on my path. Stand guard over me while I rest, and keep company with me while I sleep, protecting me from darkness. Let me remember in the depth of slumber that I am always watched over and in Your care. Shine Your grace of love and healing upon those I love and all humanity—the souls I share this journey of life with each day. I surrender my soul to this nocturnal journey, knowing that I will be returned to my body before the dawn."

Guidance: There is a healing realm of angels. Healing is their task, and it is a two-way enterprise. Heaven will not compensate for the work you must do on yourself. Heaven will not heal your darkness—that is up to you.

Intimate Conversations with the Divine human being, the grace of integrity will be given. If you ask to become more generous of heart, the grace of generosity will be poured into you. If, however, you wake with the intention to remain selfish and to deceive others, don't imagine that you have experienced a great healing. For what in you has been healed? Heaven does not let us get away with anything—but it assists us with everything we ask. Teresa of Ávila wrote extensively that the path to the soul, and thus to God, was that of self-knowledge: knowing who you are and what motivates you. You search out the dark until there is no more, and then you allow the light to speak to you. We fear the light because we think that a connection will cost us our connection with our physical life. We have this fear—and dark belief—that in order to be physical, sexual, sensual, and in touch with pleasure, we need to be in league somehow with at least a touch of darkness. We need to avoid a clear rapport with our soul lest we be conscripted into a monastery. That is all nonsense—utter nonsense. The only time I ever experience people wanting any type of spiritual intervention is when they are desperately ill. Otherwise they want to keep God 'at a distance' and their darkness mildly functional. They want to be able to hold on to 'bite-sized' dark behaviours. But conscious dark behaviour is not bite-sized. Someone is always harmed—be it yourself or someone you love—and committing conscious harm is the definition of what it means to sin. There is no such thing as a small act of darkness, just as there is no such thing as a small act of love.

Grace -The grace of Awakening is unfamiliar to people, though we often speak of it. Awakening is an experience just shy of having an epiphany—an explosion of the soul into the light.   Carolyn Myss

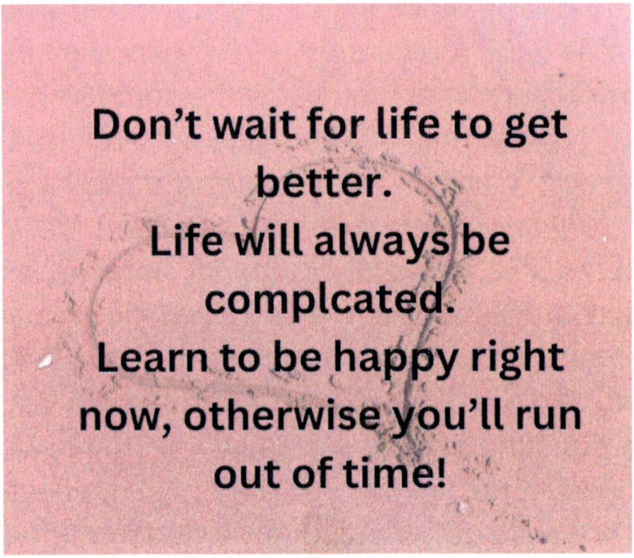

Whatever caused/created the cancer, we want to make sure we aren't repeating that pattern. So it really is about changing your vibration- really considering what do you need to do to bring joy into your life, to create more love, more happiness?

Speak words of strength and power to your body.

I AM radiant

I AM full of vigour

I AM full of energy

I AM energetic

I AM strong

I AM intelligent

I AM sweet

I AM pure

I AM wholesome

I AM whole

I AM active

I AM beautiful

I AM soft

Choose your own power words.

Ask for forgiveness from each body part for thinking they weren't these amazing qualities.

Dr Zach Bush talks about cancer being like a sprawling city taking over nature. He also says that the cancer cells are programmed to 'save you'. They believe you are dying and that they are saving you, so to change that programming, how do you convince your body that you are alive and radiant? BE alive and radiant! Dance, sing, skip, swim, hike, sit under trees, visit beaches...make a list of all the things that bring you joy and try to do at least one a day!

Make sure your list has around thirty things on it, including some that are easy and free- like dancing round the kitchen! Also have some that may cost a bit or not be so accessible but promise yourself you will do them, such as booking a massage or having a holiday. Then be sure to do one of these things EVERY DAY!!

AND have an additional list that's just twelve things- twelve things YOU REALLY WANT TO DO! These could be life ambitions; they could be your 'bucket list' things. This time it's about really doing these things and not just dreaming about them. Making plans helps us to feel we have a future to look forward to and that we will still be alive to do these things!

I always had a childhood dream of driving around the countryside in an old fashioned horse drawn gypsy wagon. In reality, I have no horse woman skills so going anywhere in a horse drawn wagon wasn't realistic. But then I realised I could just book a B&B gypsy wagon and fulfil my dream that way! So that's s what I did. We booked a little wagon on a hill side in the mountains of Wales, arranged childcare for a long weekend and off me and my hubby went. I absolutely loved it...and it shattered my fantasy of ever being able to live in such a tiny space!!

So the thing with this 'twelve things' list, is that once you achieve one of the things on your list, you add another so you always have twelve things you're planning!

Have fun with these lists. If you feel a bit blocked trying to make them, then maybe ask friends what they would put on theirs. Or just leave your list on the table and add to it in times when you're relaxed and ideas might flow. I found the more I added to my list, the more I thought of things to add!

Chapter 6

Create a new story and embrace embodiment

Cancer comes to show us things need to change; the story we are living isn't working; it's time to write a new story!

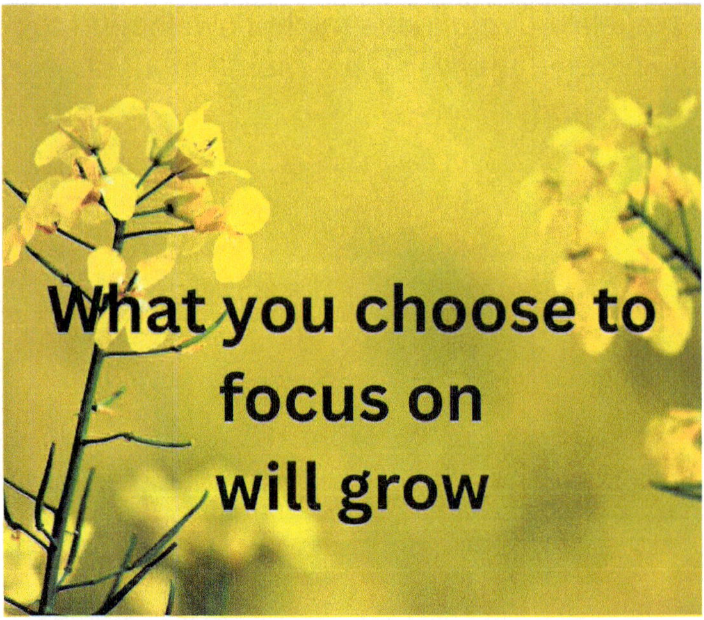

Take time to dream into your new life. I don't necessarily mean you have to move to Hawaii and spend your days drinking from fresh coconuts (but hey, that's a great dream!). Rather, what are the things you've always wanted to do/ try? We are programmed by society to work hard to pay the mortgage, get the car, have the 2.5 kids and when we retire we get to do the fun stuff. After watching my dad live this life and then die before he retired with a list of things he never got around to doing, I decided life was too short to wait to do the things I wanted to do.

Since then I've walked the Camino De Santiago, had two more children (after saying I wouldn't have any more), bought land in Wales, lived in a community, left the community, bought a yurt and ran workshops and circles, sold my business and invested in myself to do more training, booked on a week with Dr Joe Dispenza, took my children out of school to home educate, and went with my children to Harry Potter world (one on my dreams and theirs!). I now say 'yes' now when I'm invited to parties and gatherings, when I used to stay home, as I would often feel overwhelmed and shy at gatherings.

These days I enjoy the connections that happen when I push myself out of my comfort zone. I know these aren't huge things, but they were ones I really wanted to do and try. Some worked out, some didn't. But hey, I'm trying things and breaking old patterns, living life differently and making a new story of my life!

Often we can be living someone else's story without even realising it. Maybe our parents pushed us into a career before we had even decided what our interests were. Or maybe we just floated around in life, picking up whatever work came our way. Maybe we became a stay- at -home mum when really we wanted a career, or the other way around. Maybe we are carrying guilt for doing (or not doing) what we really wanted. Maybe we got married and followed our partner's dream instead of our own and lived with the resentment. Perhaps we are in a relationship that's been over for a long time but we just haven't been able to face it.

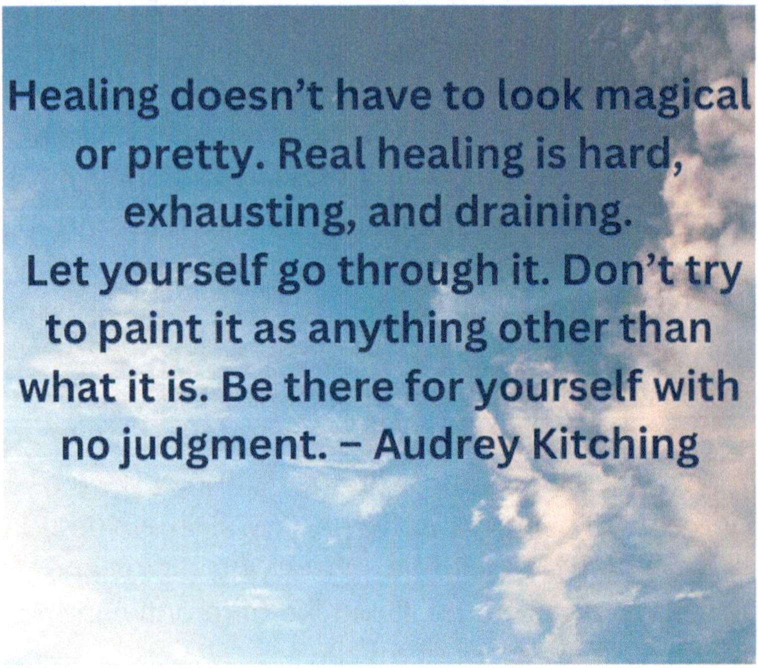

I don't know what your story is, but you do, and only you know what you need to do to change the story. And if you don't, then that's okay too; changing your story doesn't happen over night. Take time to journal, meditate, ask the Universe to show you what you need to change, or to bring you new opportunities.

Start with making a list of all the stuff that no longer serves you, and anything that causes stress in your life. What on that list can you let go? Those monthly PTA meetings- you know if you resigned someone else will take them on! The daily grind of washing up/cleaning? Can you get a dishwasher, or pay for a weekly cleaner/ ask a friend to help with cleaning while you focus on your health? Daily lifts to school; is there a friend or neighbour who can help?

For many of us, asking for help is hard, almost excruciating at times! But by not asking, we are depriving someone of the opportunity to do service in the world. Often we worry that by asking, we will cause that person to be stressed or take on too much. But you know what- that's none of your business. It's up to them to say yes or no; their boundaries are not your responsibility. And if they say no, move on and ask someone else.

Learn the mantra 'It's none of my business'.

By saying this mantra when people try and get us involved in their drama (their story!) it helps us detach and not feel as if we need to get involved. Whether it's to help or rescue. Plenty of us are good at being rescuers when, in reality this is taking on responsibility for things that are not ours, and ultimately it disempowers that person from changing themselves.

Learn to recognise what is your business (like your health, your family, and your home) and leave the rest to everyone else! When you bring this in to your life, you may notice how certain friends gossip, or are stuck in their victim story, such as telling the same problem or issue over and over but not taking advice or making any steps to change things. This can make you realise that you no longer want to partake in these scenarios. You may even notice how being around gossip and negativity affects your energy. You want to keep your vibe up, so say to yourself "it's none of my business" and walk away.

I used this mantra (along with "not my circus, not my monkeys") for a few years, and boy, did it help me shift out of unhealthy relationships and my toxic rescuer mode! I literally had to train myself each time I almost got pulled into someones drama to say to myself "this is none of my business". And as I said it to myself I would feel the weight of the responsibility to ‘fix’ or to get involved just melt away!

Like I've said before, there are always people willing to step in, it doesn't have to always be you and me.

Becoming embodied.

I had no idea what this meant until my cancer diagnosis. I think I’ve been flirting with life/death since birth. Through my teens I didn’t want to be here. I have had many attempted suicides, alongside taking drugs, drinking far too much. I made dangerous life choices. I don’t think my soul was fully incarnated. Going back and doing birth trauma work I realised I had been an unwanted baby. My mother had continued to take the contraceptive pill for the first six months of her pregnancy, denying that I was really there! Doing this birth trauma work opened my eyes to the truth of soul contracts and the contract I had made with my parents. Obviously I was meant to be here, because here I am. But on some level, none of us were sure if I would fully make it. My first suicide attempt around the age of thirteen obviously failed. I remember waking up feeling disappointed I was still here, but somehow feeling relieved. Something inside me knew that if I had died I would just be coming back and starting all over again- and the thought of going to kindergarten and primary school was enough to just keep me going!

I've recognised that I've constantly played out the story of victim, continually saying life is too much, life is overwhelming, I'm too sensitive, I feel too much. And I've also felt like I'm too much for other people; I'm too intense, I'm too serious, I'm high maintenance! Another story that needed changing- another story that was *just a story*!

So how did I become embodied? I've been studying shamanism and shamanic practices for quite a few years, doing soul retrieval, calling lost parts of myself back, but even this had not completely embodied me.

I had to make the choice did I really want to be here and, if I did, how was I going to live my life? Was I going to live it completely and fully? Because otherwise there was no point in being here.

"I call back my power" Lee Harris

And that's really how we become completely embodied; we decide to utterly and truly give ourselves to life, to absolutely accept life on this planet earth (honestly, how many times have you wanted to leave, felt it's too much, too dense, too hard here?) I realised that I had been trying to escape my body. If not with drugs, alcohol, food, or sex. Then meditation, and through books… there's so many ways to still 'numb out', even healthily!! It's about really feeling my body, enjoying my body, enjoying life, to be a full human being, earth being, Gaian, I like that name; I live on Gaia and I am a Gaian! I chose to come from spirit to experience having a body and all the amazing things a body can do; this is embodiment! I know I have repeated this over and over, but that is the key to life- to live with joy, to live in adventure, to live fully!

Chapter 7

Life beyond cancer...traversing life beyond cancer. How have I changed, what have I learnt, would I have done anything differently? What now?

Writing this book, and reflecting on this journey, would I have changed anything? When people come to me for support, I hold them in their choices which is what I have expected of my friends and my family. As for all the questioning (like should I have done this, or should I have done that?) I don't know that I would change any of my choices. Maybe I should have had surgery earlier, and possibly avoided chemotherapy. But it was all part of my journey, and through the chemotherapy I learned that I can transmute anything. I learned to surrender, and I deepened my relationships with my guides, with my angels, with my God(dess!). As well I deepened existing friendships, and made new ones along the way... and I live as a shining example of a survivor and a thriver!

As well as this, I was forced to break with the story I've been holding onto for so many years;

that allopathic medicines were poisonous, and that the chemotherapy was what eventually took my dad. Maybe it was. But that was his story and his journey, and I believe part of changing myself and changing my own story was to walk a path of natural and allopathic medicine and show that these can, in combination, be powerful and healing.

Ultimately, we choose how to heal, and I never thought I'd choose the allopathic route of surgery and chemotherapy, but I knew deep down I had to, I knew deep down it was part of my journey to accept this route and stay empowered in my own healing choices by doing what I could for myself using food, meditation, all the healing tools I had learned.

Emerging from almost a year of my life being about survival, (even though I was traversing with as much grace as I could muster). I can see it was still a year of trauma and being in fight or flight for myself and my family. At then same time, emerging from all this was just as challenging! I had sold my business, I had put ALL my focus on healing, on 'being', on upgrading myself. So now what?

How do we heal from surgery, chemo, scans; a life that's ruled by appointments, blood tests, and being poked and prodded, violated and traumatised? Life became completely saturated with appointments, healing protocols, meditation, enemas -oh the hours I spent lying on the bathroom floor!!

When all this stops, what do we do?

For me, it was by just allowing and being in the void; the place of questions, the place of rebirth and resurrection, the place of future visioning. This can be the most exciting place. Who will we be now we have been given a second chance and what will we do with it? We are reborn and get this opportunity to start over, how many of us have that? To really let go of our old life and begin anew. Who do we now want to be in the world? Who have we changed into? For we are not the same person after we've danced with death.

Yes, there's huge celebration, huge relief and the JOY of being alive. Another heart opening overwhelm of "I f**king did it!!". But at the same time, also an incubation/cocoon period.... just being in this void space..... allowing the trauma to leave, allowing the body to recover, allowing the gestation of the new self to emerge. This place is another challenge, another initiation.

It's a time of rebuilding life. I know I am changed. Facing death changed me. Surrendering over and over changed me. Choosing to let go of everything that just wasn't important for me any more changed me. My core beliefs have changed. Things that used to bother me no longer do, and things that used to feel they were vital in my life no longer feel that way. My outlook has broadened, I see things from a much more holistic place and, most surprisingly (but very much needed) somewhere along the journey I let go of the feeling I had experienced since being a child that I had to- 'fix, rescue, sort... the planet, the under dog, those in need'. The overwhelming feeling I had unconsciously carried that my 'job' here on earth was to save the planet and wake up humanity was lifted, and I felt free. I AM FREE.

Holding that gratitude every day, waking up every day with thanks for being alive, allowing that to ripple into my family, into my work, into everything my hands touch. That is the challenge.

Collectively as a world we have all, as a result of Covid, been through a huge change, a huge grief. For many of us life is not the same as it was before this pandemic. But I always knew that I was born for these times, for the change, for the building of the new, and the collapse of the old. So in some respects, it was no surprise that I had to embody the collapse of my old life and rebirth myself a new. And I'm here to show you the way; to show you that it's possible. To show you that even with a so-called terminal diagnosis you can find joy, you can find love, and you can find adventure.

How do I live now- what are my post cancer protocols?

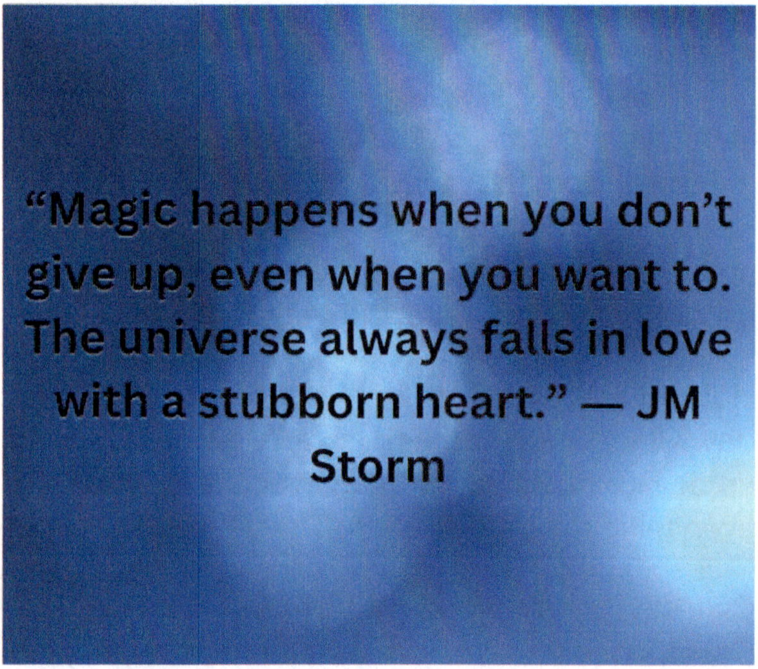
"Magic happens when you don't give up, even when you want to. The universe always falls in love with a stubborn heart." — JM Storm

So I stress here that these are my choices, and it may not be right for you. Please take responsibility for your self and your health in whatever way feels right for you.

I have chosen not to keep on going back to the doctors for regular checks and scans, partly because I know they are looking for cancer, and ultimately we all have cancer cells! So they WILL find some!!! If our body is healthy, then it knows what to do and is able to deal with those cancer cells. But if we are stagnant and not creating a good environment inside us- those cells could keep on growing and multiplying.

Self-Care Is Health Care.

My other reason for choosing to stay away from the doctors is to stay away from stress and fear. Once I had my 'all clear' I consciously chose that I was DONE with cancer.

I walked away deeply knowing I was on the golden timeline of health. I had also been on some courses with Sophie Sabbage (Cancer Whisperer) and witnessed most of those on the courses who were 'cancer free' still lived in fear of cancer returning. Not only had they put their lives on 'hold' to have treatment, they still weren't living their lives fully because of the fear of it's return. So I decided in that moment to step forward fearlessly and not to worry about cancer again.

BUT that doesn't mean I am resting on my laurels. I choose to live life fully and healthfully. I want to live a long and healthy life, so I have good daily/weekly/monthly routines. These include meditation, exercise, breath-work, and staying away from stress as much as possible. I use an infra-red lamp every other day, my itera wand daily to structure my water and realign my cells I continue to practice dowsing for health, spinning my cells, detaching from others energy, protection from EMFs and more- dowsing is magic- and fun. I also play with my singing bowls (frequency medicine) and love singing and sacred chants. I practice intermittent fasting, drink lots of water, cleanse regularly (three enemas a week- I love them!) and do a deep detox at least twice a year. I do my utmost to stay in a healthy mindset, I don't engage (much) in social media (only to promote my work- I definitely don't spend hours scrolling!). I eat from the earth. I hang out with nourishing people, and I have fun, including spending time in nature, and growing food and flowers, I do what brings me JOY! So part of this is making sure I have spa days with my girl friends, along with eating out, weekends away, as well as celebrating the holy days / holidays....living FREE and abundant.

I would also like to note that I do all this as a single mum, home educating two children. I am now post menopausal (yes all these things eased my moon- pause transition!), and I'm self employed. Believe me, if I can fit this into my life, you can too!

Of course, people say, oh well it's okay for you, I just can't fit this into my day. So I ask them; do you want to? If not, fine. But if you do, make the effort, find the time, MAKE THE TIME! I believe in divine timing; there's always enough time in the day for what's important. Plus I get up early and go to bed early.

I have learned that life is too short not to enjoy it EVERY DAY. I remember my dad saying that when he retired he wanted to walk the Camino De Santiago- but sadly he died before he retired. That was a huge wake up for me! **Don't wait to do what you want to do.** My dad's death was the catalyst for me walking the Camino and contemplating life and how I wanted to live. It was not long afterwards I had my third child and moved to Wales; it was time to start living the dream.

Chapter 8

My Healing Manifesto

How We HEAL

Live in LOVE

Create JOY in every day

Follow your INNER WISDOM

Be of SERVICE to Source and Humanity

Treat your BODY as a TEMPLE

Drink GREEN juices and eat PLANTS from the garden

Be around POSITIVITY

FORGIVE yourself and others

CLEANSE your BODY

Have a DAILY SPIRITUAL PRACTICE

Ask for HELP and call in your TRIBE

Know your ANGELS and Ancestors are with you

Meditate, visualise, have quiet moments

RELEASE old stories with EFT or TRE

BE in nature

Drink LIVE Water

CHANGE your STORY

LET GO of everything- be born anew

Say THANKYOU a lot

Talk to your CELLS- Listen to your CELLS

MOVE your body- stretch, run, dance, twirl!

ACT on your INTUITION

CHOOSE a GREAT support team of doctors and practitioners

I have a series of videos on my YouTube and my healing blog where I talk about all these points.

Since making this poster I have added a few more points. Why not make your own poster?

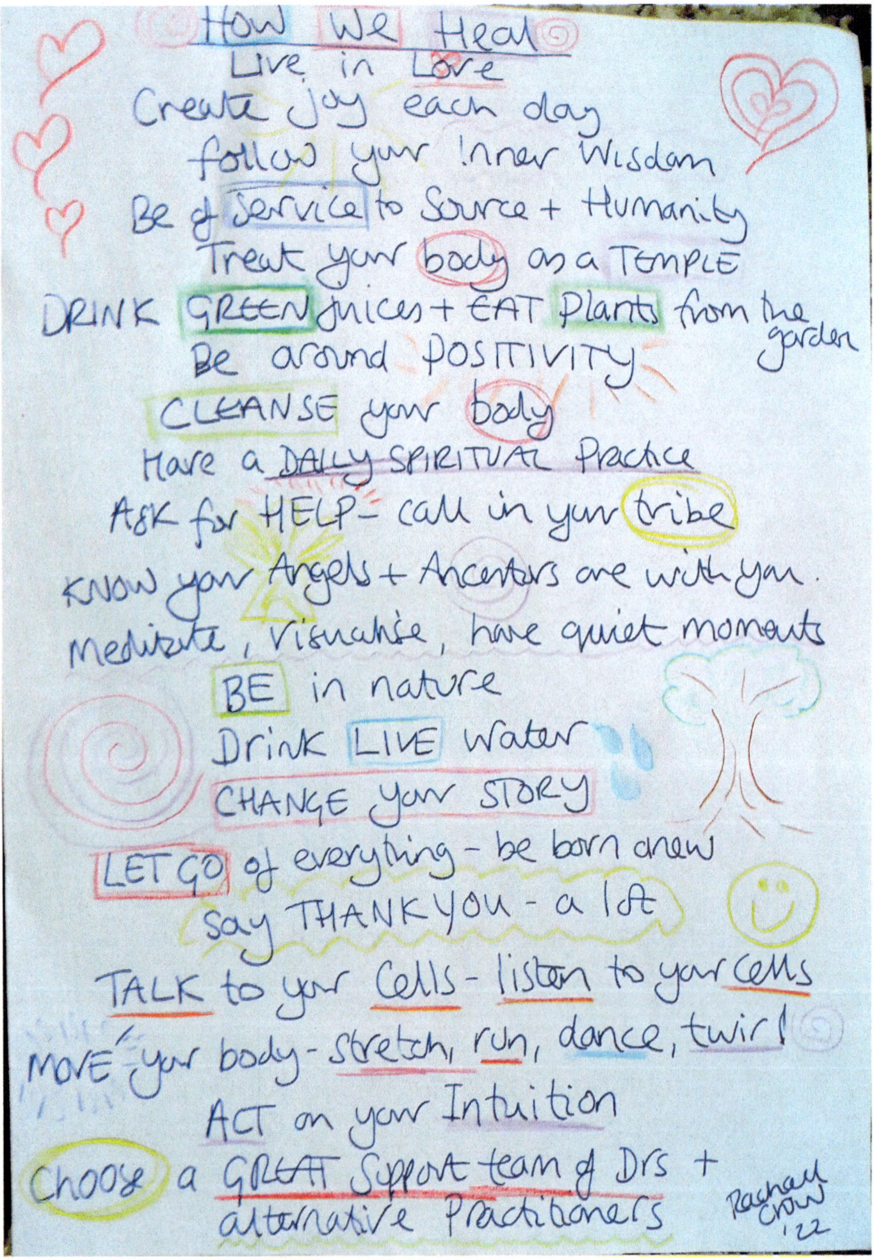

How We Heal

Live in Love

Create joy each day

follow your Inner Wisdom

Be of Service to Source + Humanity

Treat your body as a TEMPLE

DRINK GREEN juices + EAT Plants from the garden

Be around POSITIVITY

CLEANSE your body

Have a DAILY SPIRITUAL Practice

Ask for HELP – call in your tribe

KNOW your Angels + Ancestors are with you.

Meditate, visualise, have quiet moments

BE in nature

Drink LIVE water

CHANGE your STORY

LET GO of everything – be born anew

Say THANK YOU – a lot

TALK to your Cells – listen to your Cells

MOVE your body – stretch, run, dance, twirl

ACT on your Intuition

Choose a GREAT Support team of Drs + alternative Practitioners

Rachael Crow '22

Let's break these down

Live in love

What does it mean to live in love? To come to life from your heart. To ask yourself; 'what would love do now?' To prioritise loving yourself. To discover deep self-love. To do the inner work; healing work on the inner child, inner teen, inner young adult. To shine a light of love onto all the dark places, the wounds, the small hurts and love them as they are. There's nothing to change. It's just about acceptance and love. Accepting yourself wholly, and really loving yourself as the perfect being you are- even with cancer. Can you accept yourself as perfect and whole? Radiant and vibrant?

What is self-love to you? For me it's about putting yourself first, saying 'Yes' to yourself, and 'No' to others. Having boundaries. As we hold ourself in loving grace we can hold boundaries around where our energy is going; "where are you putting your energy that you could be using it to heal yourself?" If you're depleted, you need to focus on yourself. So say no to helping others, no to being around negative people/situations, no to watching the news, no to anything that doesn't bring joy into life! Surround yourself with kindness and care. Be kind to yourself, and only have people who show you kindness in your life.

No matter how difficult things are- choose love and joy! Whatever that means for you- happy music, dancing, being in nature.

In fact, grab a piece of paper right now and make a list of thirty things you love to do, from having a massage to soaking in a long bath, along with walks in nature, watching a comedy, wild swimming, a cuppa with a positive friend. Both things that cost money, things that are free. All things you can do each day and will support you in having more self-love and joy in your life!

Journal on these self-love questions; just write whatever flows....

What do you need today? How are you feeling today?

Who do you trust? What do you trust? Do you trust in your own intuition? Do you trust in your spirit guides, ancestors, angels? Can you follow the guidance of your intuition/ancestors/angels?

What do you need to let go of? What needs releasing? You could begin with decluttering, a physical letting go. Maybe there are people in your life for whom it's time to move on? Old patterns and emotions that you want to release- just be willing to let them go.

Who do you need to forgive (include yourself!)?

What do you celebrate? It's easy to find things to celebrate even when you're facing cancer- a birthday, a mile stone, a shift in the seasons or just celebrate for the sake of celebrating!!

What's important to you?

Create JOY in every day

What does joy mean to you? I didn't know what joy was until I was diagnosed with cancer. How weird is that? I would talk about joy and how I needed to have more joy in my life- but I didn't really know what joy was!

I found my joy when I decided to live life as an adventure. I decided that I would only live in joy, beauty and love- so anything outside of those parameters was OUT!! Obviously the washing up still needs to be done, so how to bring joy to that, how to bring beauty to that, how to bring love? It's all about choosing- I can choose to find washing up as joyful- I can have fun washing up, put on some music and have a little bum wiggle while washing up! I can buy really beautiful dishes that make me smile when I wash them. I can consciously send love into the water so that all my dishes give off love to all who eat from them....see?

And the irony is that I was told this by a meditation teacher when I was seventeen, but had I been unable to embody it back then. I just kept on hating the washing up!!

Really, it's about being present. Right now, I'm sitting by a river, typing this, under the sun, in a wild meadow, just after dropping my children (who are home educated) to their tutor for a couple of hours. Now, I could have gone to the near by town and mooched around the shops or sat in a cafe with the internet, but I choose to sit in nature while using my iPad to type this. This is bliss; this is how 'work' should be. This is freedom- this is joy!

It's up to you to find what brings you joy. My joy won't be your joy! So take some time right now and consider what brings you joy. Do you even know what joy feels like?

Let's try a few things. Can you remember how you felt .....

The first time you held a new born baby

Cuddling a puppy or kitten

Smelling the most delicious rose?

The moment you fell in love

Hugging someone you love

When you won something

When someone said to you 'I love you'

Dancing like no one is watching

Receiving a round of applause

I could go on. And even if most of these things haven't happened to you, can you close your eyes and imagine them? And how do you feel to imagine winning something, receiving a round of applause, a hug, dancing wildly..... hopefully you feel FREE and JOYFUL!

So keep finding ways every day to cultivate joy and your cells will thank you for it!

Follow your INNER WISDOM

I was blessed that I always had a strong sense of intuition. Even as a child I could sniff out inauthenticity a mile off- those nuns at my school didn't stand a chance with me and all my questioning of their dogma!! Haha.

I was always referred to as a 'wise child', 'old before my years', 'an old soul' and I know now deep in my bones I have been on this Earth ride many times. And yes I call it a ride as that's what its meant to be! Like choosing to go to the fair ground and getting on the big dipper as it looks so much fun, but once it starts moving we have that feeling that maybe we want to get off! Once you climb to the top and whizz down, you remember its exciting and fun- or maybe not!!! My outlook on life now, post cancer, is that were here to enjoy life. Yes, we grow through the suffering. Yes, some people have more than their fair share of suffering. But I trust there's a bigger picture. I believe we all get to 'take turns' being a goodie/ baddie, being rich/poor, living on all the different continents, in all the different cultures. In being a city slicker or an indigenous tribesman, growing up in a country of war or isolated on an island. We will get to try them all- and it's how we grow through these experiences that defines our next life- not to mention the karmic entanglements with our families and friends.

But I digress. Back to inner wisdom, although I know mine is a strong inner wisdom cultivated from many life-times here, there's no reason anyone can't learn to listen to their inner voice. Your inner voice is your higher self, your wise self, which is still connected to the Divine/God/ Source/Sophia- whatever your term might be. This inner voice will only ever be loving and reassuring. Many people ask how they know if the messages are from their higher self our just the voice in their head. Usually you can tell as most of us are highly critical with our self-talk, while our inner wisdom is only ever loving and compassionate.

I learned this exercise from a few different spiritual teachers:

Each day ask your soul what it needs.

I practiced this for many years as a womb worker, womb wise woman. I would ask my womb each day what she needed- same same, the voice of my womb is the same as my inner wisdom/higher self.

I had an interesting reaction when I was told at my first 'cancer' appointment that I would need a radical hysterectomy- I really thought that if my womb was removed I would lose my inner voice. Now I can look back and see how silly that was. But as someone who chatted to their womb every day, a hysterectomy was like cutting away my soul- and I kind of believed this was where my soul lived!!

So, another gift of having cancer was that I connected more with my whole self. I now believe this is what we are meant to be doing here on earth, embodying more and more of ourselves. Then life will just show you what you need to do.

So I realised pretty quickly that my inner voice was in fact in every cell of me, and in my energy field, and it comes though angels, guides and sometimes other people. Signs and synchronicities can be nudges from your higher self- if you're open to that!

And I want to share an insight I had after listening to a talk by Lee Harris. When he said "love is the womb of your soul", his words blew me open. It was like I had it all upside down and, back to front. My womb wasn't the place of my soul- LOVE was the womb of my soul!

So coming back to this daily practice of journaling. Asking the question- what does my soul need, or what does my body need, or what do my cells need? You will get an answer and from my experience, it is always something nourishing. My soul never suggests answering emails, or scrolling Facebook, or a coffee, or a burger. Usually it's nature connection, a juice, or a green smoothie. It can even be specific like a carrot, more root veg!! More often than not, it's to get outside, sit with a tree, go for a walk, swim in the river, anoint myself with rose oil, sit with in the rose garden, listen to Mother Earth, lie on the earth. Even though I live deep in the country-side it's really easy to disconnect myself from nature by spending too long on my laptop, and distracting myself with things to do around the house. I think we all need to make a conscious effort to get out of our boxes (houses *and* the boxes of our minds!) as much as we can. So find a daily practice that supports this Such as a nature spot to visit for five mins (or longer) each day, or a daily walk, or a run, gardening, a relaxing swing seat that entices us outside. Find a way to make being in nature easier! It's all about making things easy so we will actually do it.

Be of SERVICE to Source and Humanity

This is an interesting one, as there's a fine balance in "asking for help and receiving help" to being of service and burning yourself out. While I always advocate stopping what you are doing when you get a diagnosis, (stop work, stop mothering, stop, stop, stop) and re-evaluate your life, you can still be of service. What a dichotomy!

To simplify this: it is as basic as each morning offering yourself to the Divine/God/Source/ Whatever with the prayer

"Thy will be done".

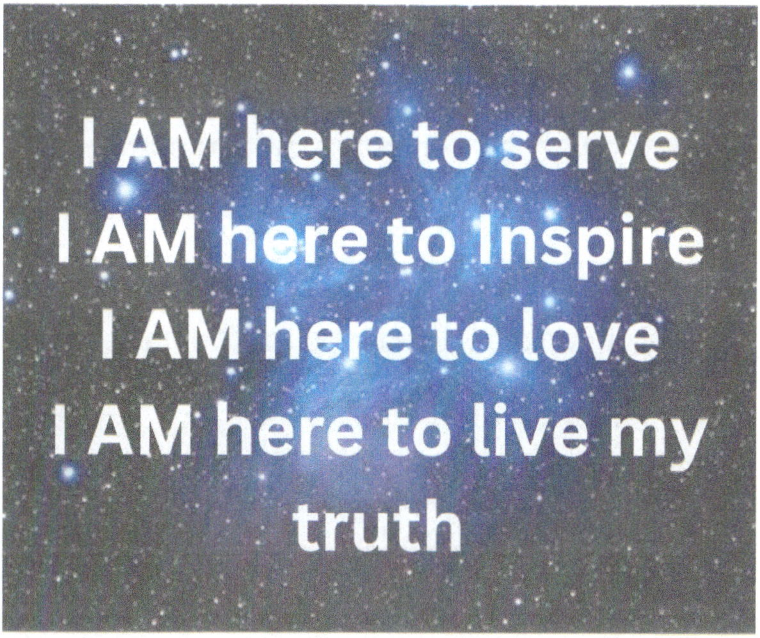

This is similar to surrendering. You're offering yourself, your life, to be of use to your Divine Source- and before you know if you will be used for *your* highest good by this Source.

Even when I was going through treatment, including the days when I could barely get out of bed, I would offer myself with this prayer. Then somehow, something would happen. Whether this was a text from someone needing a nugget of wisdom, to a beautiful email from someone who had read my blog or watched a video I'd made, thanking me for the change it had made to their life. Source knows what level of help we are able to give and NEVER asks too much of us.

So trust in this prayer - it's powerful and it brings beautiful possibilities and opportunities into your life- which in turn gives you purpose and meaning- which can be somewhat lacking when you're lying in bed not feeling able to participate much in life!!

Treat your BODY as a TEMPLE

This will mean different things to different people. I thought I already treated my body as a temple, but when I really started on my self love- self care journey I realised how much I had abused my her. I had ignored her nudges and pleas, shoved down emotions, avoided looking at past issues, shadows, and trauma....all of which are stored in our very cells.

So when I finally got it, I understood that EVERYTHING that came at my body had to be 'vetted' by my higher knowing- even down to the stuff I chose to engage with on TV, social media, and the people in my life who brought me stress. This also included the foods I ate, what I was drinking (MORE WATER- get a glass now!), exercise, self care liver wraps and enemas. For all of this, I checked in with my body- is this what I need?

If I found myself just standing in front of the fridge for no reason, I'd check in with my body. What emotions were arising? Maybe what I really needed was to do some journaling, or I needed a hug, rather than to stuff it down with food, which was an old pattern for me.

I remember at one point, when I was fasting for a few days prior to chemo I realised I had faced ALL my addictions. There was nothing left. No crutches. I just had to feel it all, let emotions flow through (mmmm, maybe cancer was partly caused by blocked emotions? I don't know but I bet that's part of it!!). And do you know what I discovered, my greatest fear was that my emotions would be too much, that they would take me over- and maybe even kill me (isn't the mind clever to plant those seeds in the psyche to keep you addicted!). And - wow- I found out they didn't! I found out that I could experience them, express them and that it was okay.I could cry, shout, rant, laugh, feel anxiety, relief, excitement, worry, sadness, grief, fear, joy, happiness .....

One of my biggest AHA moments was finding my joy.

As for the rest of it, the food and the other 'toxic' stuff, my body just doesn't want it any more! I can be around people eating cake and they say “oh don’t you want any?” Honestly, my brain goes ‘gluten, sugar, egg, dairy…ugh, NO!’

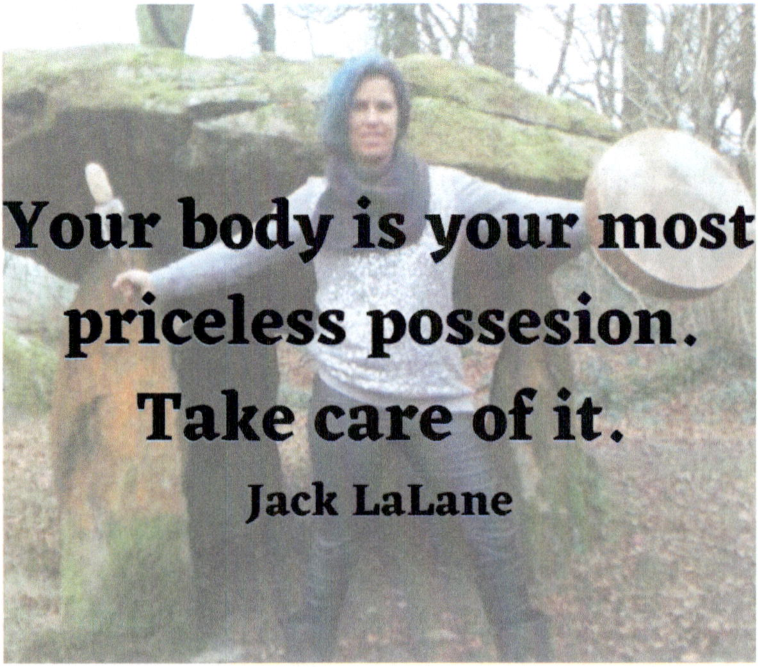

Therefore, if your body is a temple, how would you treat it? Me, I go for love, kindness, nourishing foods, plenty of water, forgiveness, constant letting go, exercise, time in nature, being around friends who bring me joy, dancing, and being creative…. The list goes on. It’s important not to become a martyr with any of this. Really do what makes your heart glow. I recently asked a friend what brings her body joy and she said ‘food’ . I checked in. “Really, does it?” (I knew she meant cake!) and she said, “honestly no, it brings me guilt.”

So, that's one to look at

Don't do things because you 'think you ought to' or out of fear. These can sneak up on you. I realised after I was all clear, that I was still taking copious amounts of supplements. My amazing nutritionist checked in with me why I was taking 'this and that' and I realised it was because they were 'anti-cancer' and I was taking them out of a fear of the cancer returning. If I truly wanted to be free of cancer, I needed to also be free of fear of cancer. Remember, what you resist persists. I had to learn to completely trust my 'all clear' diagnosis and stay cancer free by living free.

My temple LOVES FREEDOM

Drink GREEN juices and eat PLANTS from the garden

Following on from your body being your temple... FOOD! THE MOST EMOTIVE TOPIC!! I've had soooooo many conversations with cancer patients about diet, and really- no 'one' diet fits everyone. You need to listen to your body! BUT there are plenty of protocols and diets that are proven to work, and most CUT out foods known to cause cancer. Dairy and meat are the big ones, along with sugar, salts (bad ones) and processed food full of chemicals. If it's made in a laboratory it needs a laboratory to digest it (thanks Kris Carr for that quote- she's amazing, look her up). Along with fizzy drinks, alcohol (loads of sugar), starchy foods, any foods that are too acidic…

> **The emination diet - remove anger, regret, resentment, guilt, blame and worry. `then watch your health and life improve.**
>
> **Charles Glassman**

What I like to do with people I'm supporting is suggest getting all this stuff out of their diet but put their main focus on *adding* in good stuff. Basically most of what you can grow in your garden is good and the way to pack in LOTS OF IT is to JUICE IT!!

There are plenty of books with juice recipes out there. There are even companies that will deliver fresh juices to your door. I also recommend sticking to the more savoury recipes, such as green juices with lots of kale, spinach, celery. By all means add an apple or a lemon to freshen it up- but stay away from the really sweet recipes with loads of carrots, beetroot and fruits. These are all high in sugar, and whilst fruit sugar isn't the same as processed sugar, it's still best to keep those sugars LOW! Daily green juices are nutritious and filling; you will have energy, vitality and will start to GLOW! (Not green! Haha). Did you know that our body uses 80% of its energy to digest food? So by juicing we are able to use that energy to HEAL!

As well as this we need regular detoxes. We all need to detox since we live in a toxic soup. Even me who lives out in the sticks in nature, there's still pollution. Things like chemical fumes and gasses from carpets and furniture, and chemicals in clothes, and in food wrappers. Our bodies probably still have old medications floating around, things like heavy metals from vaccines, and even parasites. Yes, I mean worms, tape worms, threadworms, flatworms, round worms.... (did you know, sugar/ food cravings are caused by these parasites wanting to be fed? Best get them out!!) Ugh!

When I had cancer, I regularly detoxed and took herbs to help flush the worms out, the heavy metals, etc. These days, I do two a year- spring and autumn equinox are great times to cleanse. You can even join me as I run these online!

Make a promise to yourself to add in 1 green juice a day

Top tip: the cheapest way to do this is something like celery or cucumber and a lemon. You could add a spoon of spirulina/chlorella, be sure its all organic- no nasty pesticides!

Be around POSITIVITY

Have you noticed how negativity is much more easy to slip into than positivity?? No matter how great you might be feeling- all it takes is someone with their moaning and gossiping to bring you down to their level. So let go of those people- it's time they were no longer in your life. You need positivity while you are healing.

And yes, you could say I'm judging these people, but hey, judgment is all part of being human, isn't it?

This is about discernment, and while you're healing, creating big fat boundaries around your healing environment is important- really important.

It's not just about people- it's about everything around you. Are you living in clutter? Listening to the news, watching junk on TV? Reading low vibe novels? All of these need addressing.

I made my home my healing sanctuary. I wanted beautiful pictures, fresh flowers, pretty bedding, lightness (in all things, including light from the windows, lighter colours around me). I was constantly letting go of 'stuff'- taking things to charity shops and the charity bins in supermarket car parks. I realised I'd held on to so many things for so many silly reasons- one day this might come in useful, or twenty years ago this had cost me loads of money, or someone special gave this to me (but I've never liked it/used it.). The reasons we hold on to stuff is ridiculous! I knew if I was going to let go of cancer, I needed to let go of the 'cancerous' stuff cluttering my home. Besides, this stuff just made me feel depressed. Like the declutter queen Marie Kondo says, if it doesn't bring a feeling of joy- chuck it.

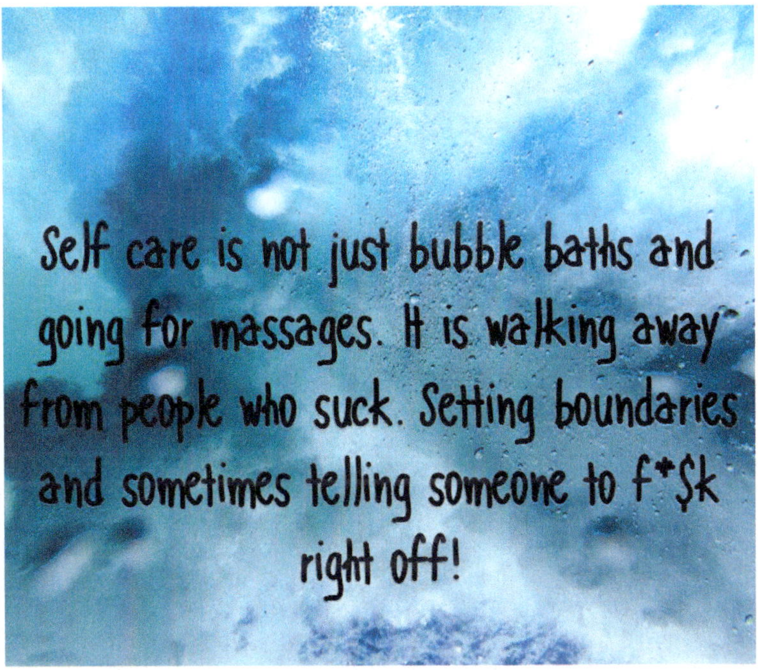

Do you listen to the news? I'm blessed I had a mother who listened to Louise Hay back in the day, and when I was around eighteen (just become a mother- feeling the weight of that responsibility on my shoulders!). She told me that

Louise Hay said not to read or listen to the news as it's energy was negative (even after all these years there's no 'positive news' channel?). So I didn't. I even made a conscious effort if I was listening to the radio, I'd turn it down when the news came on- see how sneaky they are, slotting it in to our lives every thirty minutes to keep our vibe low! We've especially seen the impact of that the last few years (2020 onwards) as fear was used as a massive weapon through the news to keep everyone doing as they were told. Over the past few years, those of us who had it all switched off and just got on with our lives have had totally different existences to the rest of the planet. My priority is always freedom; to do what supports my positive mental health and keep my children healthy and balanced.

So many people here in the UK watch the 10 o'clock news just before bed. So in the precious time that your body gets to rest and rejuvenate and heal- those pictures you saw on the news were the last thing to go into your consciousness! Or what about those people who need a radio on to fall asleep- think about what you're taking in while you're sleeping.

I recommend replacing that late night radio/news with a meditation, some relaxing breathing, a sleep visualisation, beautiful music, nature sounds- you'll sleep better and heal better!

Same for crappy TV programmes. Have you ever stopped to think about that word- programmes?

On the rare occasion I do watch something, I wonder 'what am I being programmed with?' All TV is having an effect on the subconscious. Your body is always listening, every cell is listening; so give them beautiful things to listen to. Really consider that if you love horror, thrillers, dark sci-fi, violent films, even stuff like soaps, they drop in story lines of low vibration. It's ultimately all drama and gossip- just someone else's made up drama! In fact, that's how I look at the news that does creep into my life; it's just some drama trying to pull my energy. "Not my circus, not my monkeys!"

As Dr Joe Dispenza said to me-

WHERE ARE YOU PUTTING YOUR ENERGY THAT YOU COULD BE USING TO HEAL YOURSELF?

FORGIVE yourself and others

I learned early on in my addiction recovery days that carrying resentments leads to relapse. Resentments are just old energies taking up space in our minds and our bodies. We can't help but have them; we live in a world where everyone loves to carry grudges and resentments, to moan and have things to moan about! Ultimately these negative ways of being keep us in a victim state.

I wrote earlier about how much easier it is to slip in to negativity than positivity - and that has to include our own minds.

So, how do we let go of resentments and grudges? How do we keep our minds free from negativity?

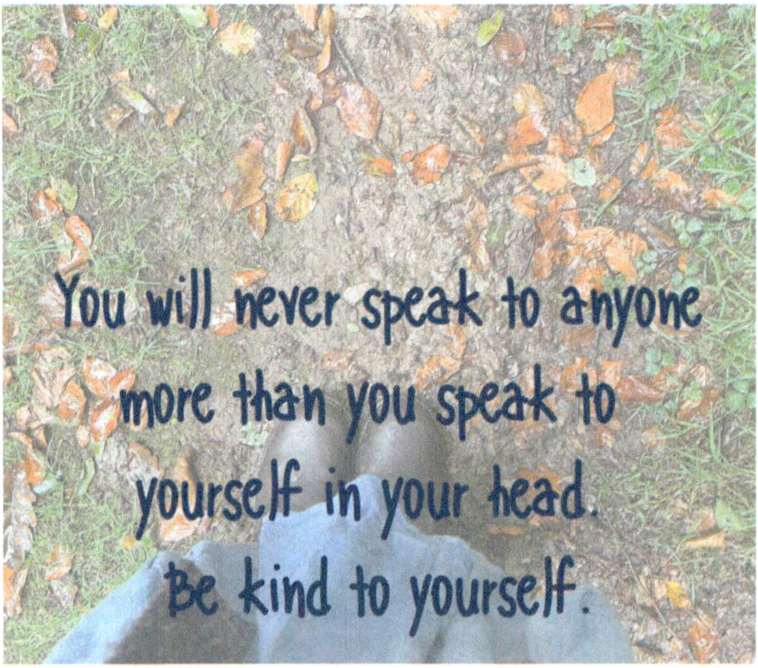
You will never speak to anyone
more than you speak to
yourself in your head.
Be kind to yourself.

First we have to have a willingness to do it. Everything has to begin with being willing to change, and willingness isn't the same as wanting to do it now. Being willing is just a small step towards that change- it's the crack in the doorway of change.

Maybe it's time to take out your journal and make a list of things you know you hold a grudge or resentment about, then sit with each one. Are you willing to let it go? Are you willing to really look at the story, and recognise that maybe, (as is often the case) it's a made up story in your mind to justify holding on? Can you release it fully? Can you forgive YOURSELF first for creating that situation and can you forgive the others involved?

Forgiveness is never about letting someone off the hook for doing something terrible- it's about FREEING yourself from holding on to that terrible thing.

Obviously, there are awful things that can happen to us when we are children, or even as young adults . Times when someone else could have protected us or maybe even the person who should have been our protector is the perpetrator. We can still find ways to forgive, to find compassion in our hearts and let go. No one hurts another person from a place of pure hatred- usually those who treat others so dreadfully have been hurt themselves.

I had some situations in my life where I was really struggling to forgive the people involved. The therapist I was working with suggested I see them as children. Of course when you imagine anyone as a child you can see their true essence, their innocence- and that somewhere along their life this was taken from them.

When it's really too hard to take the step of forgiveness, hold on to the phase 'I'm willing to forgive' and pray for help. I like to use the term 'offer it to God'. I imagine actually visiting a beautiful temple; I kneel at the altar and I lay that situation I can't deal with on the altar and let it go.

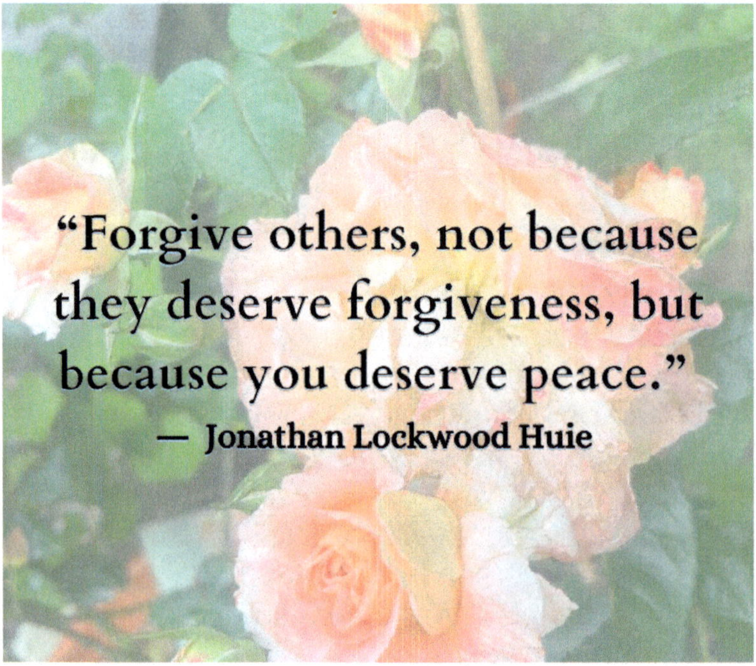

There's a saying in recovery programmes- Let Go, Let God. It just means give it all to God, and trust it will be taken care of on your behalf. The main things is that you have LET IT GO.

If this is really a struggle for you, I advise finding a counsellor or therapist you can work with.

CLEANSE your BODY Drink LIVE Water

As I mentioned earlier in the section on 'Eat plants and drink green juices', we need to cleanse. Many spiritual practices have cleansing as a large part of their physical practice. Yoga postures and breathing support cleansing and it's even written in the Dead Sea Scrolls that the Essenes like to cleanse and do enemas!

If we look around, it's not surprising we need to cleanse our bodies. Even those of us who already eat clean are up against the world of pollution in which we are all living in!

So we ALL need to cleanse- illness or not! Our bodies are struggling to process the chemicals we live in. Our poor organs are overwhelmed on a daily basis. So by cleansing, we are gifting our body a reboot.

There are many ways to cleanse, some more extreme than others. The first time you cleanse it is best done under supervision. I was blessed to have a nutritionist who offered me a place on the week of cleansing run by her school of nutrition. I did my first cleanse with them in Spain. For me it was bliss, a week of having my juices made, along with yoga every day, and group meditations, all looking at what was holding us back in life. But of course there were others who really struggled and these were the ones who needed extra support from the nutrition team, alongside the encouragement of the group. Since then I have done cleanses and fasts on my own and with other nutrition folk. I've learned so much and have plenty of tools to add to my cleansing tool box, which I now share with others on my twice yearly cleanses.

I could write loads and loads about how to cleanse here, but it's far more useful to join a cleanse and do it!

A general rule of thumb is start by taking out the 'bad stuff'. So, add more raw, greens, and salads, as well as water (good filtered /distilled water- water is life!), and juices. Alongside this, follow naturopathic techniques like liver packs and enemas (these always have to be done together), as well as skin brushing. Then, when you're comfortable with those, start eliminating solid foods and try a few days of just water and juice. Follow this by moving to just water; maybe one day of water fasting and always do enemas to support those toxins coming out of the body! Yes they can be scary at first, but I guarantee you'll end up LOVING ENEMAS!!! Hahhahaha.

I have lots of videos on my YouTube channel about cleansing and enemas.

I believe water has consciousness (highly recommend following Veda Austin and her work with water) and we are made of 70% or more water. So it makes sense to me to drink really good water, bless it, and ask it to heal, enliven, cleanse every cell as we drink it. Energise it by putting your glass over images of beauty, such as a rose, or words like love, health, radiance (you could engrave those words on your glasses- I did!), stir it/dowse it to enliven it- there's endless things you can do to bring more love into water.

Have a DAILY SPIRITUAL PRACTICE

Know your ANGELS and Ancestors are with you

Meditate, visualise, have quiet moments

BE in nature

RELEASE old stories with EFT or TRE

All these headings all come under the same umbrella for me and are the corner stone to my life and my healing journey. A deep practice of meditation, movement, gratitude, breath work and nature connection held me in my darkest moments. As I wrote about earlier, my connection to my guides, angels and ancestors got me through; I could literally feel their love and energy around me.

On the days I felt blocked and couldn't feel them, I would use my oracle cards to get a supportive message. Or I would sit in nature; find a tree to lean against and drop my 'blockages' into the earth.

I could probably write a whole book about spiritual tools to support you. You'll find plenty of information in chapter 5, as well as in the booklet that comes with the online course I put together with my friend Eartha called Initiation- Navigating the Thresholds of Illness & Death. In both the chapter and the course you'll find many tools to support you.

Your spiritual practice is just that YOURS. What works for me probably wont work for you. So find your own way. It maybe as simple as pausing before you drink your water to bless it. Or saying a little prayer on waking, and blessings the trees and plants as you walk past them. A great one is blessing the nurses, drs and those who are supporting you. Then there is gratitude for all you have (my friend Sally who had cancer in her lungs, still managed to be grateful for every breath!- how amazing is that!). Singing- even if it's just in the shower. Another one is journalling- getting all those thoughts, worries, cares down on paper and OUT of your head. Just find some way to show up for yourself and then build on it each day, spending longer and longer in the sacred moment.

It's about pushing our own boundaries, sitting in our personal practice, doing it for a little bit longer each day; taking our bodies through the FIRE of CHANGE.

There's always resistance. That's normal, we all do it. Oh I'll start tomorrow, today's not a good day. That's the body talking, the ego part of us that doesn't want to change, thats comfortable in the old ways. Well, the old ways didn't work.

It's time to take control of your life. Really it's just a game. Maybe, see it as an experiment in bringing heaven to earth? See how much joy you can create? See if you can meditate so long you get a magical experience. Do some breath work until you hit the mystical spot. THIS IS WHY we practice these things- not to be 'more holy, more spiritual', but because we enjoy the feelings and the outcome. Let's face it, who doesn't want to live a magical mystical life?

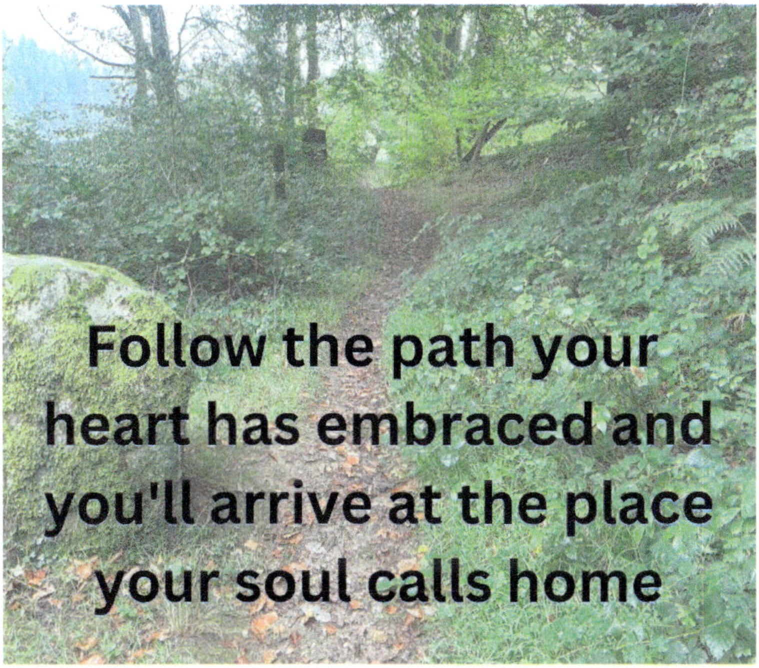
Follow the path your
heart has embraced and
you'll arrive at the place
your soul calls home

THIS IS HOW WE BECOME THE CREATOR OF OUR OWN LIFE

Releasing your old stories with EFT or TRE- now there's another section on changing your story.

But these tools are worth a mention as they can be used for SO MANY things.

Do you know about EFT? Emotional Freedom Technique is a really easy tool to learn. It's a tapping routine that stimulates the body meridians, which you can even do while driving! Haha! The therapist I went to told me that once you had the knack of the routine, you could just tap the collar bone areas and the body would remember the rest of the routine (I love SHORT CUTS like that!). So have a look on YouTube where there's plenty of videos on EFT, or book in with a therapist. Empower yourself with these skills.

TRE stands for Trauma Release Exercises. The best things to do is find a therapist offering a one day workshop. I trained with TREUK. TRE is basically shaking trauma from the body. No words, no going into story, just allowing the body to let go. I love that this is just trusting the body wisdom to do it's thing. Once you have a tool like this under your belt you can use it each time you have a doctors appointment, a scan, or any invasive treatment. Train the body to release. You can also release through dance, massage, other movement modalities. I do think years of yoga have helped me to keep the trauma of my life moving through my body. Interestingly when I was diagnosed, my yoga practice had dropped off, as had my other movement practices. Mmmm!!

Ask for HELP & call in your TRIBE

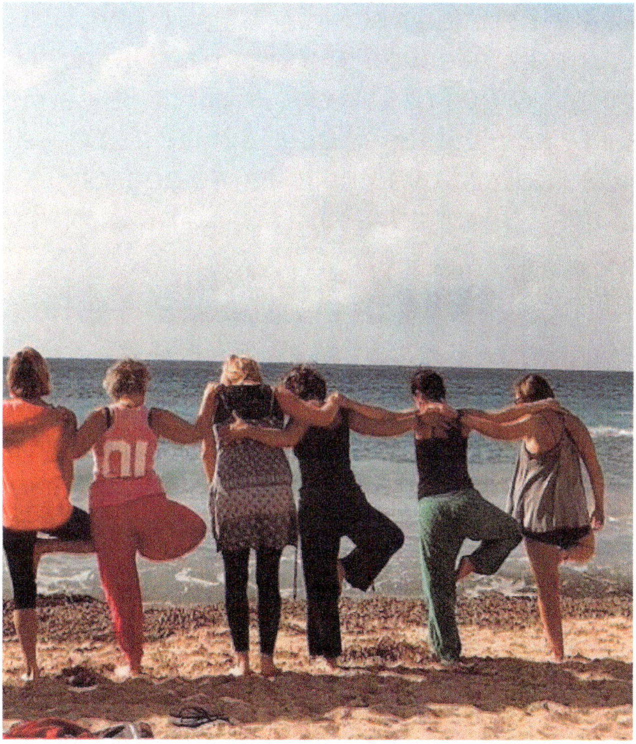

There's a saying in tribal cultures that when someone gets sick the whole tribe is grateful to that person for taking on the unconscious sickness of the village. In return, each member is part of that person's healing- and in being part of that person's healing they are witnessed and often completely recover.

This is exactly how I felt in my community. It was the hardest thing for me to do, to surrender to the fact I couldn't do it alone and ask for help.

I had always been self-sufficient. From a young age, I learned the lesson of 'no one's coming to save you, you have to save yourself'. This can be an amazing survival technique, but it does need to be broken down eventually as we actually can't do everything alone and we do need others!

Interdependency not co-dependency

My friends, along with my women's community, were awesome. They also brought in all of their skills; I had massages, reflexology, cleaning, juices and meals brought, childcare, and shamanic healings. Friends who were nurses who gave me an insider's insight as to how it might be in the hospital system. Friends (or their family members) who had positive cancer stories to share. Lifts to appointments. Friends who put me up when I travelled for treatments. The list is endless and they were all valuable.

If you are reading this as a supportive friend to someone with cancer- *anything* you can do to help will be gratefully received!

But the real healing came from me allowing in the help, allowing in the love.

LET THE LOVE IN

Opening my heart to the loving support made me realise how cut off from this part of myself I had been, and how emotionally shielded my heart had become. For when I decided I could 'do it all myself' at such a young age, I had created a barrier between myself and others. Of course the barriers would lower with certain people, such as partners and close friends, but as soon as a trigger arose, up they would go again.

I had to learn to be vulnerable and live from this beautiful heart open place of vulnerability, while also holding that strong warrior part of me that was useful now and again- but not all the time!

If this resonates with you, I encourage you to gently explore within yourself where you are too much in your self-sufficient warrior (or masculine!) and how could you let the soft, vulnerable you (your feminine) through to create balance. And then we go full circle into self-love- as ultimately being more in this loving receptive place also allows for more self-love.

CHANGE your STORY

Oh, this one can be soooo hard for people! Everyone has their victim story and the story they want to cling on to. It's the excuse they use for EVERYTHING; the excuse that blocks change. I know because I did it for years!

It’s the story that goes;

“Oh I can’t love myself because I wasn’t loved as a child….”

“I can’t change that part of myself because it’s engraved too deep in me……”

"My Cancer/PTSD/childhood trauma/abuse (add your own)..... makes it too hard....."

“I can’t do that because I have to do ….this…..first and I can’t do that until …this… changes”

“I’m like this because my parents were….”

“It’s genetic”

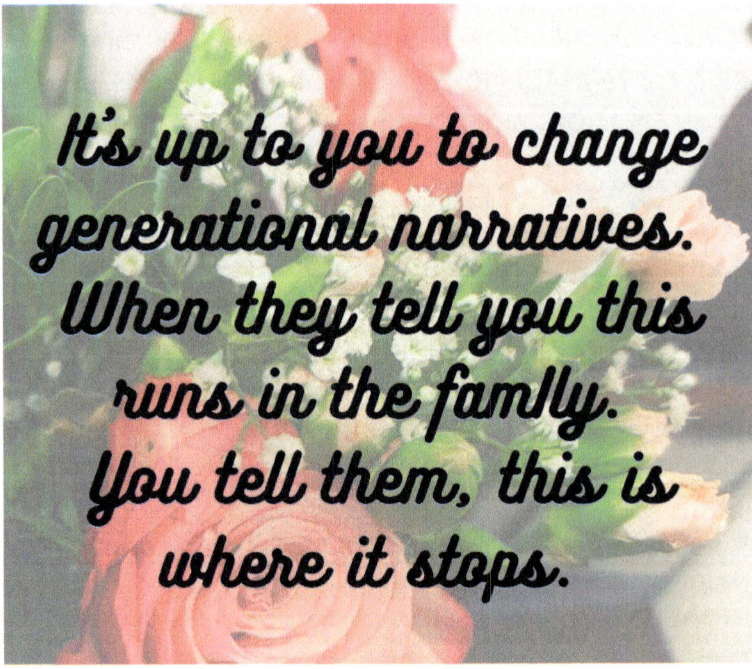

"It's just how I am"

And on and on and on....

I have seen enough people change and create miracles in their lives to know all these stories are blocks that keep us in the victim state. And yes some people love to be in that state. They love the drama, the holding on to the 'poor me' story!

It starts with- DO YOU WANT TO CHANGE?

Yes- great! Let go of the story. That's it.

Just let it go. Decide it's not going to hold you back any more!

We are so addicted to our stories, and to stress, anxiety, and drama. That's because when we constantly think about these things (such as an old resentment towards someone where you are thinking over and over about 'revenge' or what you could/should have said to them), we actually release chemicals in the body that keep us in the addiction to these emotions. Then, on top of that, we might try to 'numb out' using anything from drugs, alcohol, gaming, sex, shopping, food, the internet and social media. Guess what? We then TRAIN THE BODY to always go to that 'substance/thing' when we feel the discomfort. BUT the body will respond very cleverly. So when we get our 'hit' of dopamine from the things we use to avoid the feelings, the body goes 'oh no, too much dopamine' and actually shuts down some of our receptors. So then it takes MORE and MORE of the 'thing' to numb us and get the comfort feelings! BLIMEY! What we do to ourselves, eh?

The body loves the familiar. So we have to push ourselves out of our comfort zone of suffering and pain and practice the unfamiliar- happiness and joy!

WE HEAL THROUGH CHANGING OUR EMOTIONS

When we are addicted to negative emotions we make it really hard to change.

Like feeling angry. When we feel angry a lot, we get really good at feeling angry! When we worry a lot, we get really good at worrying. When we are anxious a lot, we get good at being anxious.

DO YOU GET IT?

So, how about practicing feeling HAPPY a lot and getting good at that? Feeling kindness a lot and getting good at practicing kindness? Feeling JOY a lot and practicing that. Then there's no need for any outside 'fixes' and you are healing yourself from your own emotions and you own body's chemistry!

YOU ARE HEALING YOURSELF FROM THE INSIDE!

And these feel-good chemicals are where the real healing happens because you are actually changing your cellular structure of the body.

So give it a go. Take a leap of faith. Believe in change, believe in miracles. BE THE CHANGE. BE THE MIRACLE. Then you can achieve ANYTHING!

My time working with chronic addicts and alcoholics showed me that anyone who really wants to change can- similar to the forgiveness. We just need to have willingness.

Notice yourself using the old excuses, catch yourself and say "no, this isn't me anymore!" I found the meditations from Dr Joe Dispenza really helpful for this, as with some of them you visualise your future self. At the end of most of the meditations he asks the question "who do you want to be when you open your eyes?" This is it, the choice point; who do you want to be? Create that version of you! In any moment, in this very moment you can be any version you want to be. Just choose it!

LET GO of everything- be born anew

Similar to choosing to let go of your 'story' (whatever that is), you can choose to COMPLETELY SURRENDER and let go of life.

Really, this is facing death fully and surrendering to 'what will be'. Whilst this can be scary (and perhaps feel we are inviting death in), it really is how we free ourselves.

In the willingness to completely release ourselves from life and death, we become free to choose to live!

I became a bit obsessed with being 'baptised'. Not in the religious sense, or as part of being 'baptised into' something like a church, or into Jesus' life, but to be baptised INTO LIFE! I explored this for quite a few months, even chatting to a branch of Christians who did baptisms in rivers and at the beach. But there was a catch "you have to give your life to Jesus afterwards" Erm…no, thats not what I'm looking for!

I was blessed to have the opportunity to baptise myself when the week before I was due to have surgery I had my moon blood come. I knew this would be my last ever bleed and I wanted to honour it in some way. I felt giving it back to Mother Earth and her blood was the ideal celebration. So I called the women, we went to the river near my home. We circled, burned sage, and made prayers. They painted my body with ochre and I got in the river and plunged myself, with the intention that the 'me' that came out of that river was reborn. I was Rachael v.2, a new me, one that was being given a second chance at life.

And I was!

I believe its time we reclaimed these words and traditions and make them our own. Baptism, resurrection, anointing…these are all things we can undertake without priests, and vicars, and those who see themselves as the 'only line to God'. We have the power to have divine revelation. We just have to follow our intuition and feelings; they will always lead us on the right path.

Say THANK YOU a lot

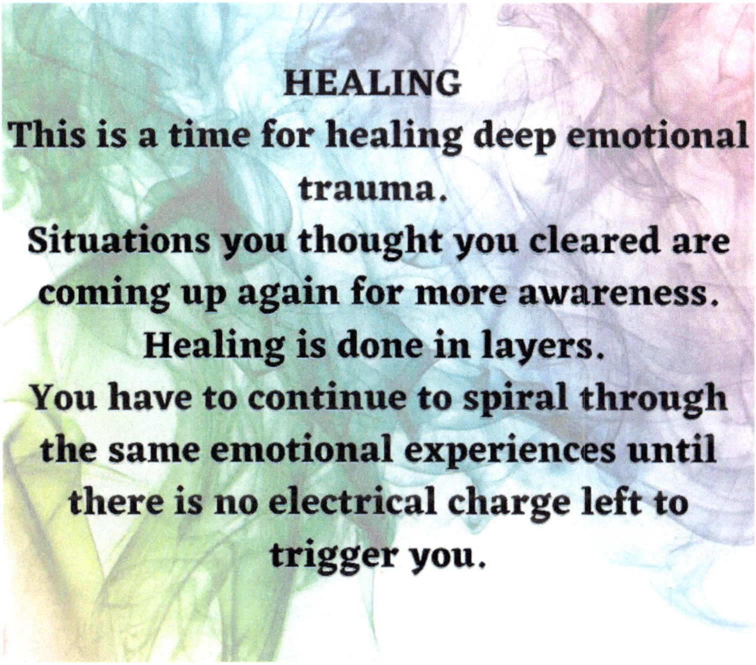

There have been whole books written about gratitude, abundance, and the heart opening, life opening magic that happens when you bring gratitude into your life. It's interesting that the more you bring it in, the more you will notice others who don't!

Not that you need to pay that any attention, but when you're used to saying thank you and being in gratitude its very noticeable when people don't respond back with gratitude. Again, it may be time to let those folk slip away.

Once you begin on the journey of gratitude, you will become addicted and notice fast results. You feel happier, and the universe reflects the gratitude back by creating more things for you to be grateful for.

All through my allopathic cancer journey I was grateful over and over for appointment cancellations and the times when treatments couldn't happen for various reasons. Others in a similar situation were panicking; they NEEDED the appointment, the scan, the treatment, and they needed it NOW! But if you slip into DIVINE TIMING and TRUST, then in pops gratitude. I was sooooo grateful I had more time for my own healing choices, to add in more green juices, another acupuncture session, more rest, more time with my children....

It was a HUGE LESSON in GOING WITH THE FLOW

At every step I trusted the Universe was working in my favour and if something got changed or cancelled I said thank you. I knew there was a bigger picture going on that was helpful.

So start every morning waking in gratitude for another day on Planet Earth.

Be thankful for your amazing body.

Be grateful for your friends and family, cats and dogs- whoever you live with and is around you on a daily basis.

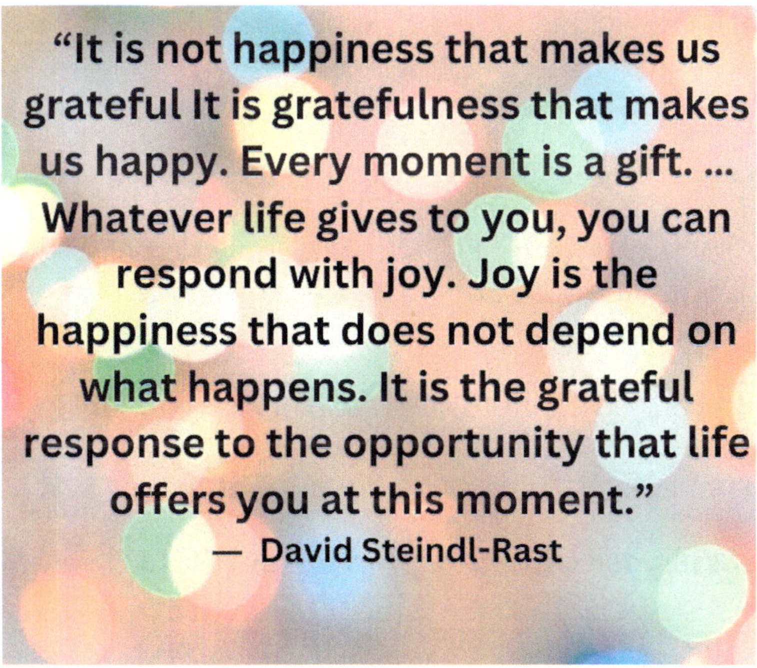

Be thankful for the food you eat- and gratitude to all the folk who were part of the chain from planting the seeds to getting it to your mouth.

Be thankful for your home, your healing temple.

Give gratitude for enough money to pay for everything you need.

Be grateful for the car/bus/taxi/bike that transports you around.

Be grateful for the inspiring people around you.

Be thankful for the help others offer.

Be soooo grateful for nature in all its beauty and for the delicious food and sustenance Mother Earth provides.

Be thankful for clean water and a power supply to you home.

I could go on and on…Take time now to make your gratitude list and make daily gratitude part of your daily journaling .

End your day, before you sleep, listing everything you are grateful for and leave a note by your bed to remind you to practice gratitude.

Talk to your CELLS- Listen to your CELLS

I almost feel like I could teach a class on 'channelling messages from your body' because this is kind of what talking to your cells starts- a whole amazing conversation with your body!

I wonder if you've ever spoken to a part of your body before? I named my blog 'Hello Cervix' as I felt I'd ignored my cervix all the years I'd taught womb work, but of course I've also ignored my little toe, my elbow, my fingernails- haha!

It's time to see your body as a whole- every cell in communication with all the others. One of the amazing facts I learnt on the many nutrition courses I've followed was that when a single cell is cut off through dis-ease, high cholesterol, or illness, it is no longer in communication with the other cell 'buddies'. If lots of cells are sick- wow there's a whole lot of 'no-communication' going on. And we also mirror that on the outside by feeling cut off, depressed, and low! So it's VITAL we support our cells- and one step is to talk to them!

It may feel weird at first (in fact I pretty much guarantee it will feel weird!) but you'll be amazed at what answers come though when you get into deep conversation with your cells. And don't censor it; don't push it away saying it's just your imagination, especially if what's coming though is good stuff. All our cells want is to bring radiance, vitality and coherence to our bodies- even the cancer cells.

Start by just placing your hands on your body and saying hello, and I bet they will be overjoyed to have connection with you. Maybe write out some questions for them:

Hello cells, what do you need today?

What will help you today?

What will support both of us today? (yes you may feel a little schizophrenic but who cares if you get some inner wisdom!)

What will bring you into balance and radiance?

You can ask deeper questions, but be prepared for what may come as an answer.

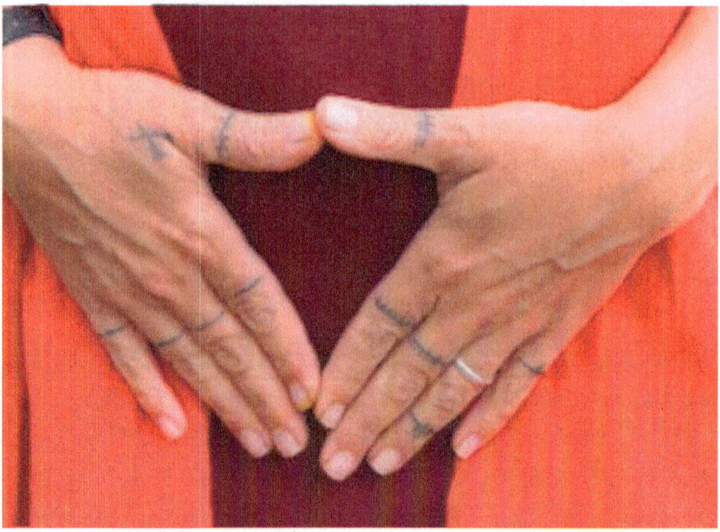

Why are you sick?

Why have you become cancer cells?

What do I need to learn from this?

TRUST what comes through YOU.

It's really useful to have a buddy to listen to your answers. If not, then read them out loud, and read them several times over during your healing journey. There's something powerful about hearing your own body wisdom out loud and I believe there is MAGIC and POWER in the spoken word.

This is how Jesus healed; he ordered those bodies to heal with firm conviction. If we order our cells to be vibrant, radiant, balanced and coherent every day, every hour, in every moment- we will heal!

MOVE your body- stretch, run, dance, twirl!

Your body is made to MOVE!

Most folk live VERY sedentary lives. We go from bed, to the table, to the car, to the desk, back to the car, the sofa and bed. It's no wonder we have dis-ease!!

Find ways to move your body that are easy, achievable and FUN!

I didn't realise how much I did move until my children signed up to walk up Kilimanjaro as a sponsored walk. We were walking up local hills, our own stairs, and in woods, measuring each time until we reached the same as the height of Kilimanjaro! Well, once I spent a day counting how many times I ran up stairs I let myself off the hook with exercise! Although I did have a rebounder for jumping on to get my lymph going, and I would on occasion jump on the trampoline in the garden with the kids (great pelvic floor work out!!), and eventually I found the Couch to 5K app and started running and discovered I LOVE running! I can also be found dancing round the living room for some extra heart pumping exercise!

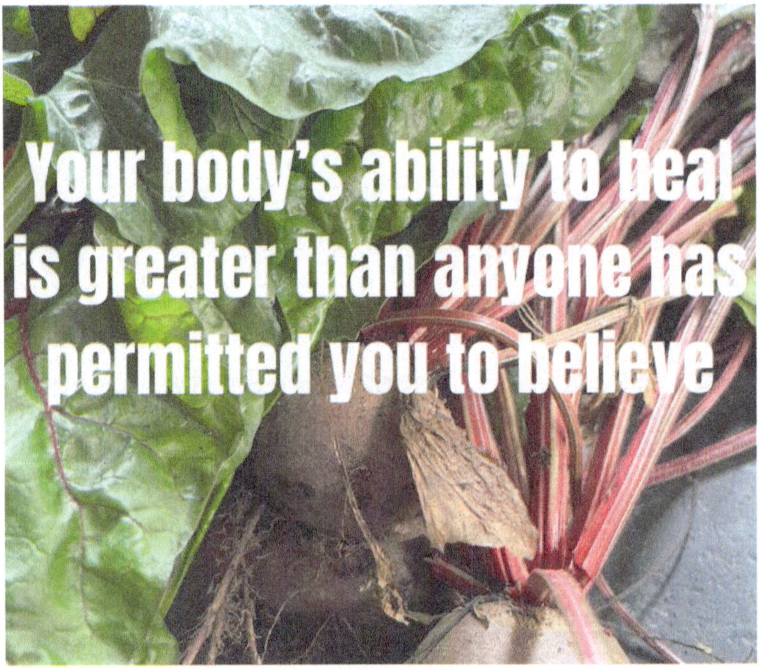
Your body's ability to heal
is greater than anyone has
permitted you to believe

GOOD MUSIC helps (and you could dress up!). With all these things, our bodies love music, so make yourself a play list of uplifting good dance tunes (remember that positivity vibe- no broken hearted love songs) and get your body moving to those.

Lastly try skipping- when did you last skip? You can't help but laugh when you skip. It takes you right back to childhood. I think there's even someone I saw online who started a skipping movement. How much more fun would life be if we were all skipping down the road?!

ACT on your INTUITION

I've talked OVER AND OVER about following your intuition, your gut feelings. It takes courage to totally trust those inner nudges and act on them, but I promise you they will pay off.

There were many, many times I thought I was going bonkers. I questioned what I was doing, and why I was doing it. But as I sit here today, typing this, almost three years since my surgery. I can say with my hand on my heart I wouldn't change any of it.

I empowered MYSELF by following my own inner truth.

I healed MYSELF by following my inner compass.

I DID IT MY WAY! And I believe thats why I'm alive today. No one coerced me, bullied me, feared me into anything. I prayed, I asked for guidance, I surrendered and trusted- over and over and over...

And I knew deep down I would have a miracle. That I would be a miracle. And so every day I felt like a miracle!

Today I still feel like a miracle- totally blessed to be alive.

I AM A MIRACLE

CHOOSE a GREAT support team of doctors and practitioners

Finally, and maybe this should be first, but I think it takes time to build your team…

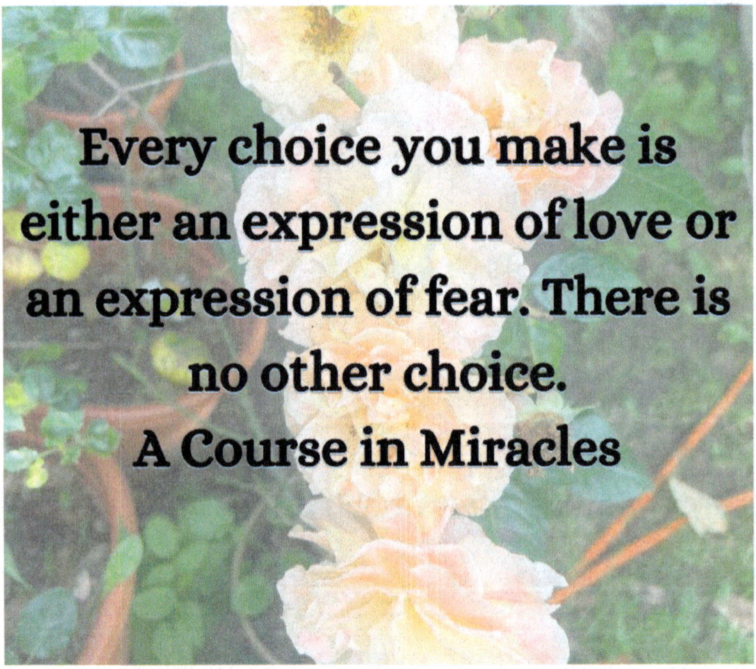

You're entitled to a second opinion. To ask for another doctor, to ask to be referred to someone else if you need it (remember to use your angelic guidance and ask them to bring the right people to you).

If any of the doctors or practitioners suggest things you're not happy with, tell them. They are there for YOU not the other way around. You're in charge.

I worked with many natural practitioners along-side my doctors. I also have an anthroposophical doctor in Stroud who prescribed and administered mistletoe, she would also look at my scan results and wanted to be involved in treatment discussions.

Here are some of the practitioners I worked with

Naturopath/nutritionist

Herbalist

Bio Hacker (he would also do blood tests)

Acupuncturist

Colonic Practitioner

Massage Therapist

Shamanic Practitioners

Psychotherapist

Cancer Mentor

Homeopath

Kinesiologist

Reiki practitioners

Energy healers

Channellers

Psychics

PLUS, all my amazing friends who gave me cranial, reflexology, neck rubs, foot rubs, and just spend time chatting to me, checking in on me, coming for a cuppa.

NEVER UNDERESTIMATE the power of a cuppa and a chat.

So there we are. This is my story and suggestions for you in a nut shell.

Ultimately your journey is your journey. You have to go it alone, that's what an initiation is. You can do it. And even if you die trying- that's the next big initiation waiting for us all. And there's no failure in death. It's the one guarantee in life- so live your life as fully as you can.

Much love and JOY, Rachael

25th July 2023. A Day Out of Time.

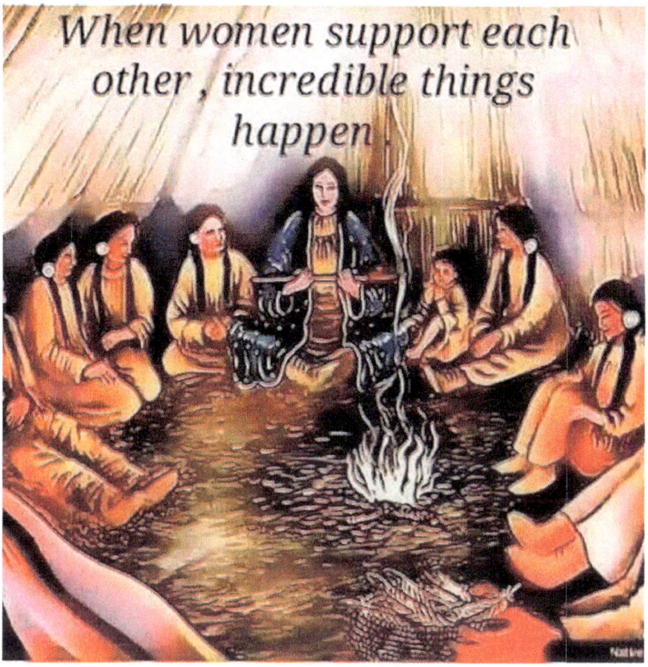

My Healing Prayers and Affirmations

As with all the other tools I have shared, prayers too need to be spoken with conviction and feeling. Really FEEL the love of the Divine, and KNOW She is supporting you. And yes, sometimes we have to fake it to make it! Keep practicing! Prayers need to be embodied in to every cell. Choose your favourite (or what you need in this moment) and make it your healing mantra.

I give thanks that my life forces are vital and radiant.

I give thanks for the orderly adjustment of every function of my body.

I AM strengthened, renewed, whole.

I AM a radiant child of the Divine

My mind, body and affairs NOW express divine radiant perfection.

I forgive everything, everyone, every experience, every memory of the past or present that needs forgiveness. I forgive positively everyone. The Divine is love, and I am forgiven and I am governed by the Love of the Divine. Her love is now adjusting my life and its problems. Realising this, I abide in peace.

I am Divine intelligence: every part of my body is filled with divine intelligence. I am whole, well and harmonious, through and through.

I praise my body as a prefect creation of Divine bounty now.

Let there be health and wholeness in my mind and body now.

I now let go everything and everybody of the past or present that has caused discomfort in, through or around me. We all go free to greater wholeness.

There is nothing to fear, for there is no power to hurt or be hurt in this situation.

The Aramaic Lord's Prayer

O Birther! Father-Mother of the Cosmos

you create all that moves in light.

Focus your light within us, make it useful:

as the rays of a beacon show the way.

Create your reign of unity now,

through our fiery hearts and willing hands.

Your one desire then acts with ours, as in all light, so in all forms.

Grant what we need each day in bread and insight:

subsistence for the call of growing life.

Loose the cords of mistakes binding us,

as we release the strands we hold of others' guilt.

Don't let us enter forgetfulness,

But free us from unripeness,

From you is born all ruling will, the power and the life to do,

the song that beautifies all, from age to age it renews.

Truly, power to these statements,

may they be the source from which all my actions grow.

Sealed in trust and faith. Amen.

Prayer of St Francis

Lord, make me an instrument of Your peace;

Where there is hatred, let me sow love;

Where there is injury, pardon;

Where there is doubt, faith;

Where there is despair, hope;

Where there is darkness, light;

And where there is sadness, joy.

O Divine One,

Grant that I may not so much seek

To be consoled as to console;

To be understood, as to understand;

To be loved, as to love;

For it is in giving that we receive,

It is in pardoning that we are pardoned,

And it is in dying that we are born to Eternal Life.

Amen.

Mother Mary full of grace, holds me safe within her eternal embrace.

My Queen and my Mother,

I give myself entirely to you;

and to show my devotion to you,

I consecrate to you this day my eyes,

my ears, my mouth, my heart,

my whole being without reserve.

Wherefore, good Mother,

as I am your own,

keep me, guard me,

as your property and possession.

Amen.

Holy Mary,

help those in need,

give strength to the weak,

comfort the sorrowful,

pray for God's people,

assist all who are In need.

Mary may all who seek your help

experience your unfailing protection. Amen.

Mary, health of the sick, you brought forth into our world Jesus Christ, our Divine Healer. In your caring goodness, intercede for those with cancer who are truly in need of miraculous assistance.

If it be God's will, I ask this day that the gift of healing from all forms of cancer be granted to everyone. Comfort them during times of anguish, pain, confusion and despair. Ask our gracious Saviour to grant physical health, inner peace and patience to those suffering.

May God's healing graces grant us a life of happiness, health and fulfilment here on earth. Amen

Hail Mary, full of grace, the Lord is with thee.

Blessed art thou among women, and blessed is the fruit of thy womb

Holy Mary, Mother of God, pray for us

now and at the hour of our death. Amen.

Speak words of strength and power to your body.

I AM radiant

I AM full of vigour

I AM full of energy

I AM energetic

I AM strong

I AM intelligent

I AM sweet

I AM pure

I AM wholesome

I AM whole

I AM active

I AM beautiful

I AM soft

Choose your own power words.

Ask for forgiveness from each body part for thinking they weren't these amazing qualities.

Book recommendations-

The Magic - Rhonda Byrne

When the Body says No - Gabor Mate

The Secret C - J A Stokes(for children)

Overcoming Cancer - Walter Last

Chris Beat Cancer and The Square One healing cancer coaching programme - Chris Walk

The Cancer Whisperer and Lifeshocks - Sophie Sabbage

Cancer and the New Biology of Water - Dr Thomas Cowen

The Metabolic Approach to Cancer - Dr Natasha Winters

Gerson Therapy - Charlotte Gerson

Herbal Medical Healing and Cancer - Donald Yance

Cancer, Why we are still dying to know the truth -Phillip Day

Radical Remission - Kelly Turner

Mums not Having Chemo - Laura Bond

Crazy Sexy Cancer – Kris Carr

Cancer As a Turning Point: A Handbook for People with Cancer - Lawrence Leshan

The Dynamic Laws of Healing - Catherine Ponder

A Year to Live - Stephen Levine

You Can Conquer Cancer - Ian Gawler

You Can Heal Your Life - Louise Hay

Fat for Fuel Ketogenic Cookbook: Recipes and Ketogenic Keys to Health - Dr Joseph Mercola

Down There - Susun Weed

My Videos and Courses

My blog https://tinyurl.com/2e8pf2fs

My post op video https://tinyurl.com/26c9927d

Body of the earth video https://tinyurl.com/3cax6y5c

Post Lletz Trauma https://tinyurl.com/3v8aya5s

My Mary Magdalene on line course where I share my Golden Body story https://tinyurl.com/yc2hr67d

My video diaries from the Dr Joe week https://tinyurl.com/49u9txpv

My series of videos on my healing manifesto https://tinyurl.com/2vfmhwh4

Cancer as an Initiation- accompaniment course

This course includes loads of resources such as foods for those starting on the healing journey, simple recipes, herbal allies, care packages, what books to read, which cancer influencers to follow, videos, meditations, rituals to incorporate around allopathic treatments/scans, how to step away from the fear and scanxiety.

PLUS my my DEEP detox programme worth £55

https://tinyurl.com/mpkxdaam

Cleanse with me!

https://tinyurl.com/yhsjcr5y

Navigating the thresholds of Illness & Death - mini course where you'll find many tools to support you https://tinyurl.com/3anchena

About me!

I am Rachael....My life's work and purpose is to empower people to awaken to their authentic powerful self.

Originally a Liverpudlian, I settled and raised my two eldest children in Bristol, before moving out of the city with my husband and third child to 'live the good life' in West Wales. I now have four children and live deep in magical countryside surrounded by trees, rivers, lush green meadows, and standing stones with my youngest two who we co-parent and home educate.

Primarily I am a mother but also a Teacher of metaphysics/spiritual tools, Workshop Facilitator, doula, breastfeeding mother supporter, artist, Medicine Drum Maker, Massage Therapist (including womb and fertility massage) and Reiki

Master/teacher. I have run Red Tents and Moon Lodges for over thirty years, I've written articles for magazines such as Kindred Spirit, Juno and Aeva (previously She Who Knows) and a number of blogs.

I spent many years as the manageress and creatress of Moon Times eco femme wear company.

I've been on a path of transformation since my late teens when I became interested in meditation, intuition and self-healing. I studied self growth, mysticism and metaphysics from a young age. I was initiated by Isis when I was nineteen and pregnant with my second child. She opened me to remembering my past life as a temple priestess and has put many of my past life soul group into my path. In 1999 I hit a 'rock bottom' with addictions that opened me in a way I never thought possible. I know now this was due to my Saturn return, and having a 'peak experience/kundalini awakening', that brought a massive spiritual opening.

Since then I've been able to see the world from a different perspective, and so, hold a vision of a bigger picture, and work with angels, guides and spirit animals. Since this time I have been in recovery from alcohol and drug addiction, food issues and co-dependency.

Each day I have offer myself in service to Spirit and Mother Earth and every day is an adventure. In 2018 I was diagnosed with cancer. Again, this opened me to another level of awakening, more 'peak experiences', and opening even more to the Divine and her love for humankind. I had no fear of cancer and only trusted this was another level of healing for me. As Anita Moojani says "Cancer came to save me!" I journeyed the healing path for three years, alongside supporting others on their healing journeys, bringing in love where there is fear, light where there is darkness. To support my peri menopause and cancer journey, I practised meditation, breath work, yoga, reiki, conscious cycle charting, Trauma Release Exercises, nutrition, naturopathic techniques and other natural healthy ways of living and healing. I'm trained in holistic massage, womb massage, womb healing, reiki and yoga.

I love to be in nature and walk everyday in the beautiful surroundings of my home.

I have been inspired by and worked with many amazing women and men over the years. I've also worked in the voluntary sector with women with addictions, as well as a drugs worker, counsellor and a community artist.

I spent a couple of years on the holding group of a Sufi camp that we attended as a family for many years and embraced Dances of Universal Peace (dances and songs of many traditions, many Aramaic and Hebrew), Sufi practices and working with the Aramaic Lords Prayer. (see the work of Neil Douglas Klotz).

For over twenty years I have worked with individuals, groups and communities; offering workshops and classes such as: Reiki Classes, Workshops; Thirteen Moons year-long training, 'Celebrating Menarche'- mother and daughter days, rites of passage ceremonies with young women, 'Gifts of the Menstrual Cycle' menstrual awareness courses, Womb healing sessions (in person and distantly) and in my doula work I offered blessingways and naming ceremonies.

I am particularly passionate about working with women at their transitions- Menarche (first blood), Mother/ birthing yourself as a Mother, Honouring hysterectomy, infertility, peri menopause and menopause. I even fundraised to create a real life Red Tent for women to gather in during their moon time! I love bringing people to the heart beat of our Earth Mother, to quieten ourselves and deeply listen to her messages, through our wombs, drum journeys, nature connection....We can all pause, breathe, drop our roots down and connect to the earth any time and listen to her wisdom.

I am Earth Keeper, I am the earth, I hold the earth at my centre and consider her in all my actions.

As part of my healing I joined Perdita Finn, Strand Clarke and many others in these Way of The Rose circles Praying the Rosary together... taking me back to my past temple life once more – igniting a deeper longing to be with my sisters in prayer.

I am dedicated to my own journey of self growth and to supporting others on theirs.

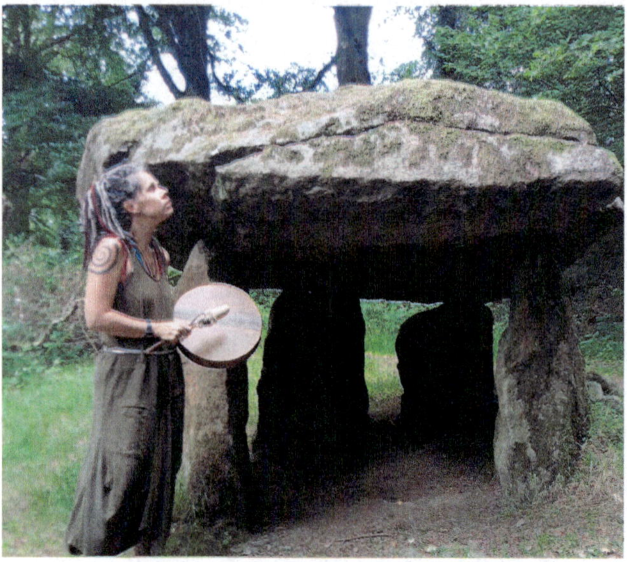

Glossary

Abraham Hicks: A popular spiritual and self-help teaching series based on the teachings of Esther and Jerry Hicks, often focused on the Law of Attraction and manifestation.

Acupuncturist: A healthcare practitioner specialising in acupuncture, a traditionalChinese medicine practice involving the insertion of fine needles into specific points on the body to promote healing and balance.

Affirmations: Positive statements or phrases used to promote self-belief and positive thinking.

Allopathic System: The conventional medical approach to treating diseases and health conditions, often involving the use of pharmaceutical drugs and surgery.

Anaesthetist: A medical professional who specialises in administering anaesthesia and monitoring a patient's vital signs during surgery or medical procedures.

Biopsy: A medical procedure that involves the removal and examination of a small tissue sample to determine the presence of cancer or other diseases.

Blood Tests: Laboratory examinations of blood samples to assess various health parameters, such as cell counts and biochemical markers.

Bowel Removal: Surgical procedure involving the partial or complete removal of the intestine (bowel) due to medical conditions, often requiring a stoma (an artificial opening for waste elimination).

Brandon Bay Journey: A self-help and healing approach developed by Brandon Bays, involving emotional release and personal transformation.

Cancer Diagnosis: The determination of the presence and characteristics of cancer, often involving medical tests and examinations.

Catheter: A medical device used to drain urine from the bladder when normal urination is not possible, often inserted through the urethra or abdominal wall.

Chemo/Radiotherapy: Cancer treatments involving chemotherapy (drug-based treatment) and radiotherapy (radiation-based treatment) to target and destroy cancer cells.

Collective Story: A shared narrative or belief system held by society or a community.

Cocoon: A symbol of seclusion or introspection, akin to a chrysalis in which transformation occurs before emerging as a butterfly.

Community: A group of people who provide support, care, and a sense of belonging.

Dark Nights of the Soul: Periods of intense emotional or spiritual turmoil, where one confronts their inner struggles and undergoes profound inner change.

Divine: Often used to refer to a higher power or spiritual force guiding one's life.

Divine Plan: A belief or concept that suggests life events are guided or influenced by a higher power or cosmic order.

Enemas: A procedure used to introduce liquids into the rectum and colon for various purposes, such as cleansing, medication administration, or hydration.

Exploratory Examinations: Medical procedures performed during surgery to assess the extent of disease or abnormalities in the body.

Empowerment: The process of gaining the confidence and ability to make one's own decisions and choices.

Five Elements: In traditional Chinese medicine, the five elements (wood, fire, earth, metal, and water) represent various aspects of the body, mind, and emotions and their interconnectedness.

Flower Essence Consultation: The use of flower essences, such as Bach flower remedies, to address emotional and psychological well-being.

"F*!k Cancer": A phrase often used to express defiance and determination in the face of a cancer diagnosis.

Gratitude: A feeling of thankfulness and appreciation for the blessings and support in one's life.

Gynaecologist: A medical doctor who specialises in the female reproductive system, including the diagnosis and treatment of conditions related to the uterus, ovaries, and cervix.

Healing: The process of recovering from illness or injury, both physically, emotionally and spiritually.

Hysterectomy: Surgical removal of the uterus, a common procedure for the treatment of various gynecological conditions, including cancer.

Incarnate:In the context of spiritual belief, it refers to the act of a soul taking on a physical human form for a specific lifetime or experience.

Inner Healing: The process of healing emotional, psychological, or spiritual aspects of oneself.

Initiation: A ceremonial or symbolic introduction to a new experience, knowledge, or responsibility, often associated with personal growth and transformation.

Intuition:A person's ability to understand or know something without the need for conscious reasoning, often seen as a form of inner guidance.

Internal Checks: Medical examinations or tests that involve an assessment of internal organs, often used for the diagnosis and monitoring of health conditions.

Joe Dispenza Retreat: A retreat or workshop led by Dr. Joe Dispenza, a prominent figure in the field of meditation, healing, and personal transformation.

Juicing: A dietary practice that involves extracting juice from fruits and vegetables as a way to consume essential nutrients.

Life Initiations: Significant life events or transitions that lead to personal growth and self-discovery, often celebrated through ceremonies or rituals.

Liver Packs: A therapeutic technique that may involve applying warm compresses or packs to the liver area to support liver health and function.

Lymph Nodes: Small, bean-shaped structures in the lymphatic system that play a role in filtering and fighting infections.

Matrilineal Line: The ancestral line or lineage through one's mother or maternal side of the family.

Medicine Pouch: A small pouch containing symbolic or power items used for healing, protection, and personal empowerment.

Meditation: A mental practice aimed at relaxation, focus, and inner peace, often used for stress reduction and mental well-being.

Metastasized Cervical Cancer: Cervical cancer that has spread to other parts of the body, typically through the lymphatic system or the bloodstream.

Mistletoe Injections: A form of complementary and alternative medicine involving the use of mistletoe extract to treat various medical conditions, including cancer.

Nudges, Shoves, Shouts: Metaphorical stages of increasing urgency in the messages life sends, encouraging personal growth and change.

Oracle Cards: Decks of cards used for divination or as tools for personal insight and guidance.

Ovarian Cysts: Fluid-filled sacs that can develop on or within the ovaries.

Palliative Care: Medical and supportive care focused on improving the quality of life and providing comfort for patients with serious or terminal illnesses.

Reflection: The process of looking inward and examining one's life, choices, and experiences.

Re-Staged: The process of reevaluating the extent and severity of cancer after additional diagnostic tests or procedures, resulting in a new stage classification.

Recovery: The process of regaining one's health, well-being, or a sense of normalcy after facing a challenging situation, such as a cancer diagnosis.

Resilience: The ability to adapt and cope with adversity and challenging situations.

Rites and Ceremonies: Formal and symbolic rituals or activities, often associated with transitions or significant events.

Rites of Passage: Ceremonies or rituals marking transitions in life, often associated with significant milestones or changes.

Scans: Diagnostic procedures that use imaging techniques, such as ultrasound

Smudging :Smudging is seen as a way to restore balance and harmony, clear negative influences, and connect with the spiritual realm. It is used in various contexts, including personal purification, preparing a sacred space for meditation or ceremony, or cleansing a new home.

Printed in Great Britain
by Amazon

53140350R00126